THE FEMALE HEART

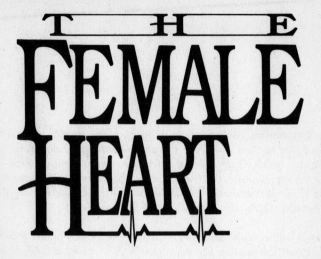

THE FEMALE HEART

THE TRUTH ABOUT WOMEN AND HEART DISEASE

MARIANNE J. LEGATO, M.D.,
AND CAROL COLMAN

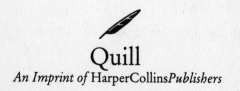

Quill
An Imprint of HarperCollinsPublishers

A hardcover edition of this book was originally published by Simon & Schuster in 1991. It was first published in paperback by Avon Books in 1993. It is here reprinted by arrangement with Simon & Schuster.

HarperCollins books may be purchased for educational, business, or sales promotional use. For information please write: Special Markets Department, Harper-Collins Publishers Inc., 10 East 53rd Street, New York, NY 10022.

First Quill edition published 2000.

Library of Congress Cataloging-in-Publication Data has been applied for.

ISBN 0-688-18065-5 (pbk.)

00 01 02 03 04 RRD 10 9 8 7 6 5 4 3 2

To *Justin* and *Christiana*
M.L.

To *Joshua* and *Michael*
C.C.

ACKNOWLEDGMENTS

MANY people helped us with this book. We'd like to thank Marianne
Sciberras, M.A., R.D., for her advice on nutrition. We would also like
to thank Patricio Paez, M.D., and Margaret Chesney, Ph.D., of the
University of California at San Francisco for their help with the chapter
on women and stress; Dan Myers, director, Health and Fitness Services
for the 92nd Street Y, Lars G. Ekelund, M.D., Ph.D., and Steven Blair,
Ph.D., for providing information on exercise; and Jack Slater, M.D., of
New York University for giving us a historical perspective on cardiology.

Much thanks to Stephan Sorrell, M.D., director of the substance
abuse program at St. Lukes–Roosevelt Medical Center, for his insights
on women and addictions, and to Steven S. Khan, M.D., of Cedars-
Sinai Medical Center and the UCLA School of Medicine, Los Angeles,
for reviewing his work on sexual bias in the referral of women for bypass
surgery. We'd also like to thank the staff of the American Heart Association for the prompt attention that they gave our inquiries and a special
thanks to Cindy Burns at the New York chapter for all her help through
the years.

We owe a special debt of gratitude to our editors at Simon & Schuster,
Marilyn Abraham and Sheila Curry, for their help in making this project
a reality. Carol would like to thank her brother, David Colman, Ph.D.,
for answering all her questions, and her husband, Michael, for his help
on this and other projects. We also want to thank our agent, Richard
Curtis, for his support in this and all our other endeavors. Most of all,
we would like to thank Dr. Legato's students and patients for teaching
us so much about what we have written.

CONTENTS

PREFACE

In the six years since Carol Colman and I wrote *The Female Heart*, society's interest in women's health has exploded. Until the late 1980s, two thirds of all research on diseases that affect men and women equally was done exclusively in men. By 1992, the National Institutes of Health (NIH) mandated that females be included in clinical investigations wherever appropriate. The Federal Drug Administration (FDA) followed suit, making drug testing in women mandatory for approval of new medicines that were intended for use in both sexes. As a result, scientists made tremendous progress in learning more about the female patient. Cardiovascular disease was no exception; in fact, we've refined and expanded our ideas about how coronary artery disease affects women to the point that our work in cardiology is a model for scientists working in other specialties of medicine.

Relying on experimental data harvested from studies in men to decide how to care for women is no longer acceptable; females aren't just small males but have a unique physiology we must understand if we are going to save women's lives. We're using the new gender-specific information to correct our male models of normal human function and of how individual diseases actually work to cause disability and premature death.

The National Institutes of Health has just finished a landmark survey of what we know about female biology.[1] The report, sponsored by the Office of Research on Women's Health, includes a list of the most important new directions for future research on women.

Here's some of what we've learned about women and coronary artery disease since *The Female Heart* was first published.

The numbers of people with coronary artery disease has decreased 2 percent a year since 1980. Only 29 percent of the decline is due to fewer risk factors for CAD in the population; the rest of the decreased incidence is due to improvements in treatment. However, Americans are living longer, so that the absolute numbers of patients with CAD

1. "Beyond Hunt Valley: Research on Women's Health for the 21st Century," *Report of the National Institutes of Health*, Office of Research on Women's Health, National Institutes of Health, Bethesda, MD, forthcoming.

has increased. They are having a more chronic form of the disease. If we're going to have any success in lowering the incidence of the disease (and mitigating its severity), we'll have to improve the population's risk factors.

That's going to be hard to achieve; doctors aren't doing a very good job in counseling women about their risk factors for CAD. We did a survey of women in 1997; they told us what happened when they went to their physicians for their checkups. We learned that doctors counseled men about how to prevent heart disease more than they did women. Not surprisingly, cardiologists were the most likely (and gynecologists the least likely) to discuss prevention of CAD with their patients. Women said that 59 percent of doctors don't talk to them at all about heart disease, only half check their patients' cholesterol value, and 87 percent don't take the time to measure the waist-hip ratios of their patients. As for women themselves, 44 percent of women believed they were unlikely to have a heart attack in their lifetimes, and 56 percent believed their risk for breast cancer was the same or greater than their risk for CAD.

The discussion about whether or not to take hormones after menopause continues, but it's easier now to make a decision about what's right for the individual patient. Research about estrogen and the way it acts in the bodies of both men and women has produced a rich yield of very important new information. Estrogen is not just a reproductive hormone—it has more than 400 sites of action in the body and is an important growth and repair agent for all the tissues and organs of the body. Estrogen users have a lower incidence of Alzheimer's disease and only half the CAD that's present in nonusers. There are studies now showing that estrogen stabilizes the coronary arteries and prevents spasm in both women *and* men, and recent work shows that estrogen may be helpful in the treatment of men with coronary artery disease, just as it is in women. New compounds, called "designer" estrogens or SERMS (selective estrogen receptor modulators), are being developed: tamoxifen was the first and a new drug, raloxifene, has just been released. These compounds react with tissue receptors in some, but not all, of the organs in which estrogen has an effect. That gives women a wider choice of hormonelike compounds that can produce some of estrogen's good actions (like prevention of osteoporosis) without some of its less desirable side effects. Raloxifene, for example, works as well on bone as does estrogen, but doesn't stimulate breast tissue or the uterine lining, so that women using raloxifene don't have to use progestrone to prevent endometrial cancer. There may be some real drawbacks to these new compounds, though: some women complain of "fuzzy thinking" and memory loss on raloxifene and tamoxifen. These "designer estrogens" may, in fact, be blocking the effect of estrogen in the brain, where that hormone works to maintain neurons in good repair and working order. We need much more long-term experience with these newer drugs.

The new data, though, shows that estrogen doesn't simply work to prevent osteoporosis and coronary artery disease. It's also important for maintenance of intellectual function, for prevention of diseases of the urinary tract (including frequent infections and urinary incontinence) and for maintaining a good sex life. Not only does estrogen help prevent vaginal thinning and dryness, which makes intercourse painful, but it works to keep orgasm intense and easily attainable for women who notice that their sexual pleasure is less than it was when they were pre-menopausal. Other benefits of estrogen include thicker, less dry, and less wrinkled skin as well as flexible and less painful joints.

We've made progress in research looking at the reversal of coronary artery disease in both men and women. Dean Ornish's recent observations suggest that coronary artery plaque can actually regress with careful and consistent treatment in both genders, but that therapy is more successful in this regard in women. Women show other benefits with treatment that men don't enjoy, too: they are less likely to restenosis coronary arteries after angioplasty than are men and, as equally aggressive treatment is being offered to men and women for CAD, mortality with interventions like coronary artery bypass surgery is no longer higher in women than in men, as was the case previously. Earlier diagnosis and more aggressive treatment for women have improved the dreadful statistic that showed that white women were twice as likely to die as white men after their first heart attack: recent studies have suggested that the death rates are now about equal in both genders.

Important new questions are being asked now: doctors are trying to understand and unravel the correlation between stress and cardiovascular disease. Patients have always understood that stress exacts a toll on the heart; scientists are trying to find out exactly now this happens. The results of stress are different in men and women in important ways, though: males feel anxiety about their jobs, but women are more likely to worry about failures in personal relationships. It may also be true that the heart's vulnerability to pressure may vary as a function of gender. For example, a threat in the outside world causes a chain of events in the brain, pituitary, and adrenal gland. The result is that the adrenal secretes "stress" hormones that ready the human for retaliative action. One of these hormones is cortisol. Cortisol works to soften the stress reaction and inhibits the impulses in the hypothalamus and pituitary that "turn on" the adrenal gland. In women, estrogen seems to diminish the effect of cortisol on the stress response, making a threat have more lasting effect in the female than in the male. More research is needed to understand the differences in men and women in this important and poorly understood area of cardiovascular medicine.

New tests are available now for detecting coronary artery disease. One of the latest is the ultrafast CAT scan of the coronary arteries, which detects calcium in the vessels even before symptoms of the disease become apparent. The test, equally accurate in men and women, is useful in patients at high risk for developing coronary disease but in whom conventional testing is negative. Interventions have improved, too: balloon angioplasty, or percutaneous transluminal coronary angioplasty (PTCA), done in combination with irradiation of the lining of the affected coronary makes restenosis less likely.

In short, we continue to press ahead with new and exciting information about how to prevent, ameliorate, and even reverse coronary artery disease. We still have a monumental educational task ahead, though, which is to tell physicians and patients alike just how important the new information is and to translate the latest science into less virulent, less frequent disease. I'll know I've succeeded when our next survey shows that doctors are counseling all women (and men) about how to prevent coronary artery disease from early adult life onward, when women and men are receiving equally aggressive therapy for CAD, and when women answer when I ask them what disease they fear most not "breast cancer," but "heart disease." We hope *The Female Heart* will help with that work.

Marianne J. Legato, M.D.
September 30, 1998
New York City

INTRODUCTION

WOMEN AND HEART DISEASE: A CASE OF NEGLECT

WHEN people ask me why I decided to write a book on women and heart disease I tell them about my friends, Ted, a physician, and his wife, Janet. Last year, Ted and Janet, both forty-eight, were vacationing at a small New England resort. One morning, Janet woke up with searing chest pain that persisted on and off throughout the day. Both she and her husband assumed she had indigestion.

The next day, when Ted and Janet were hiking in the woods, Ted complained of chest pain. Both Janet and Ted were terrified that he was having a heart attack. They quickly returned to the hotel and called a local doctor who instructed them to go immediately to the hospital emergency room. There Ted was given a battery of tests and the doctors discovered that he had an acute inflammation of the covering of the heart caused by a viral infection. Only later that day did Janet remember her own chest pain and mention it to the emergency room physician. He then tested Janet's blood and, sure enough discovered that she too was suffering from the identical heart problem. Despite the dramatic symptoms, the condition was not very serious, and resolved on its own.

Here is a case of two people, one a physician, who had identical symptoms yet they responded to their own and each other's problem in completely different ways. No one, not even Janet herself, regarded her pain as serious enough to warrant calling a doctor. The possibility that something might be wrong with her heart was the farthest thing from her mind, not to mention Ted's. But when Ted complained of chest pain, both Janet and he had the same first thought: *heart attack*! And their second thought was to get him to a doctor quickly. As I listened to Janet tell this story some weeks later, it was amazing to me that even as she told it, she still did not see the disaster that might have been caused by her neglect. In fact, her own illness had been diagnosed only by accident!

I am a physician who teaches, practices medicine, and does cardiac research in New York City. I can tell you that in all of these settings I have seen different versions of Janet's story repeated time and time again, sometimes with disastrous consequences. The possibility that women might ever suffer a heart attack is so far removed from most women's minds that they usually do nothing to lower their risk of heart disease, and they usually seek treatment long after they should.

Why? I think this attitude reflects a belief held by many men and women—physicians and laymen alike—that heart attacks are solely a "man's problem."

Most heart attacks are caused by coronary artery disease (CAD), a condition that occurs when the arteries feeding blood to the heart become narrowed or blocked entirely. CAD is an equal opportunity killer. It is the leading cause of death of both men and women in the United States. Despite this fact, my women patients are far more worried about cancer. While it's true that 40,000 women die of breast cancer each year, 250,000 will die of a heart attack. Considering these statistics, I am always amazed that without exception all my women patients have gynecologists; "going to the gyno" is routine for them. Yet none of them worries about heart attack. This is not surprising: neither does most of the medical establishment!

For many years, even researchers believed that the female lifestyle or female hormones protected women from CAD. However, we know that women—both homemakers and those who work outside the home—are subjected to as much stress as men are, or more. Moreover, we know that a woman's so-called "hormonal protection" is merely a postponement. After menopause, a woman's risk of heart disease rises dramatically with each passing year. Although heart disease typically strikes women about ten years later than it strikes men, in many ways it is far more devastating for women. If a woman gets a heart attack, she is twice as likely to die from it as a man, and is twice as likely to have a second attack. Medical researchers now suspect that CAD progresses more quickly and is more lethal in women than in men, since half of females (compared to only one in four males) die of their first heart attack.

Ted and Janet's story also reflects the fact that a woman's cardiac symptoms are not taken as seriously as a man's—not even by the woman herself. Janet was lucky that she was not having a heart attack. Many women who experience similar bouts of chest pain *are* having heart attacks, but like Janet they dismiss the pain as trivial. Incredible as it may seem, the fact is that about 35 percent of all heart attacks in women go unnoticed or unreported!

Not only are women guilty of minimizing their task of CAD but so are many of their doctors. A recent study done at Einstein College of Medicine in New York reveals that cardiologists are much more likely to dismiss a woman's symptoms as "noncardiac" than they are a man's. They are three times more likely to diagnose a woman's chest pain as being "in her head" as they are a man's. The study also showed that doctors are ten times more likely to refer male CAD patients for further testing than female patients to determine whether surgery or other treatment is possible. Another study done at Cedars-Sinai Medical Center in Los Angeles suggested that the delay in diagnosis and treatment of women may be responsible for the fact that women are nearly twice as likely to die during coronary bypass surgery than men.

This abounding ignorance about the female heart is not surprising. The overwhelming majority of cardiac research has focused on men. Nearly every major study—ranging from an investigation of the benefits of eating fatty fish to the pros and cons of taking aspirin to prevent heart attack—has involved male patients only. Today, less than 20 percent of the research budget of the National Institutes of Health is spent on women's health. As a result, the need for information about disease in women has become so pressing that in 1986 the National Institutes of Health made a formal plea for scientists to include women in research study populations. This plea was only a suggestion—not a requirement— for winning federal funds. Recently, the NIH issued a statement warning that if women are not adequately represented in any research proposal it might compromise the funding of the project. It is a step in the right direction, but unfortunately, it may be years before we reap any benefits from this new policy.

The information obtained from studies that exclude women does not necessarily apply to women. Men and women are biologically different, and as a result, the course and treatment of heart disease in men and women are different. There is one major study that did include women and has given us a wealth of information. Begun in 1948, and known as the Framingham study, this project has followed the lives of more than 6,000 men and women living in a small New England town, focusing on heart and blood vessel disease in general, but principally on the causes, course, and treatment of CAD. Since it is one of the few major studies to include women, and to alert us to the special dangers of CAD in females, we refer to the Framingham studies quite often throughout this book.

My coauthor Carol Colman knows only too well how symptoms of heart disease in women can be neglected by patients themselves and by their physicians. When she approached me to collaborate on this book, she told me about her mother's experiences with cardiovascular disease. In 1965, Carol's mother, Ruth, was diagnosed as having extremely high blood pressure, or hypertension.

"High blood pressure is known as "the silent killer," because its victims, have few, if any, symptoms, at least early in the disease. Yet, if untreated, high blood pressure can lead to heart attack, stroke, and kidney disease. Since Ruth was symptom-free, she simply ignored the diagnosis. Within a few years, however, she began to slow down considerably. The slightest exertion left her breathless and exhausted, which is often a sign of a failing heart. At that point, Ruth went to a doctor who prescribed a diuretic (a pill that helps rid the body of salt and water) to reduce the blood pressure. The medication didn't work, and Ruth sought help from another doctor who put her on a different medication. Ruth's pressure was still high. When she asked her doctor if there was anything else that could be done, he said no. He told her, quite correctly, that in 95 percent of all cases the cause of hypertension is unknown, and therefore, there was no reason to look any further. When she continued to complain of excessive fatigue, her doctor began talking about "housewife's blues."

Ruth's stamina continued to deteriorate and she began to spend more time in bed than out of it. Carol pleaded with Ruth to see another doctor, but Ruth refused. Even Carol's brother, David, a medical researcher, could not budge her. Ruth acknowledges, in retrospect, that she was afraid to seek another opinion for fear of finding out that something else—perhaps something more serious—was wrong. Finally, a family friend, a woman medical student, dragged Ruth screaming, if not kicking, to another internist. The new doctor listened very carefully as Ruth described her symptoms and then he proceeded to do a thorough examination. Among other things, he discovered that a kidney problem was causing her high blood pressure, that she had an underactive thyroid gland that was causing some of her fatigue, and that her heart had been damaged by the combination of the two. Because he listened carefully to Ruth, and did not dismiss her complaints as hysterical, the doctor was able to treat Ruth very successfully.

Within a short time, she was a different woman, literally full of life and bursting with energy. The woman who had once had difficulty getting out of bed in the morning was able to get a part-time job and lead a normal, active life.

Carol is convinced that had her mother not agreed to be seen by another doctor, her diseases would have killed her. I think Carol is probably right. Although Ruth has done amazingly well considering the circumstances, she paid dearly for neglecting her health all those years. Five years ago, she developed an arrhythmia and needed a pacemaker to help regulate her heartbeat. Last year, Ruth suffered a small stroke. From her mother's experiences, Carol learned an important lesson. Like so many other women, Carol once believed that heart disease was a man's problem. Now she knows that even her own heart is vulnerable.

Carol and I wrote this book to alert women to heart disease: how it affects them, what they can do to prevent it, and most important, to warn women that they are not immune to CAD. We also explain how the normal functioning of the female heart is different in important ways from that of a man. Women's unique biology puts special demands on the heart, not only during pregnancy and menopause but during the ordinary course of their reproductive lives.

This book is not solely about the biology of the heart. A good doctor treats the entire patient: heart, body, and soul. We are not just a collection of cells and chemicals. Our well-being and indeed our eventual survival depend on a whole constellation of things: What happens to one part of the body often has an effect on another part. The lives we lead can have profound consequences for our mental and physical well-being. It's important for a doctor to get to know her patient as a person, just as it is important for a patient to realize that her lifestyle can also affect her health. That is why this book is not just about arteries, veins, and ventricles. It is about how women live and about how, by taking better care of their hearts and themselves, they can improve and extend their lives.

I

THE HEALTHY HEART: WHEN THINGS ARE GOING RIGHT

❧

Chapter 1

THE NORMAL FEMALE HEART
AND HOW IT WORKS

THE alarm clock goes off half an hour late and you have to be in the office at 9 A.M. sharp for a special meeting with the head of your division. You jump into the shower, gulp down your coffee, and get dressed in record time. You're in luck—the baby sitter is only five minutes late! You run to your car and race to the train station to catch the 8:10. Just as you pull into the jammed parking lot, the train pulls into the station. You frantically search for an empty space. You manage to find one. The train doors open and people begin to pile in. You grab your briefcase and start to run. You hear the conductor shout: "All aboard." You run even faster down the long, narrow platform. You know you can make it! You throw yourself into the last car just as the doors begin to shut. Exhausted and out of breath, you sink into the first available seat. Your palms are sweating. Your blood pressure is soaring. Your heart is pounding away at 160 beats per minute, which is nearly twice its normal rate. You sit. In a few minutes you stop panting and your pulse returns to normal. But then your mind begins to wander. You begin to think about the presentation you will be giving to your colleagues later that morning. At the mere thought of speaking in public, your stomach churns with anxiety. Your heart begins to race inside your chest. It beats faster and faster. . . .

It's all in a day's work for your heart, an amazing muscle that in most cases meets whatever physical and psychic challenges life doles out to it and to its owner. It will take tremendous abuse, but, as you will see, even this miraculous organ has its limits.

Long before scientists understood the function of the heart, people intuitively sensed the crucial role it played in sustaining life. Since the earliest days of recorded history, the heart has been endowed with metaphysical powers. In ancient Egypt, the fate of the soul was thought to be determined by the weight of the heart. Egyptian priests used to weigh the heart of the dead on a scale against a feather, in the belief that those who had hearts that were not "heavy with sin" went on to happiness in the afterlife. The great philosopher Aristotle

3

thought that the heart was the seat of the soul, and attributed mystical powers to this hardworking muscle.

Even in modern times, the mere mention of the word *heart* conjures up images of love, romance, and emotion. We think with our brains, but we feel with our hearts. Our romanticized image of the heart is reflected in the traditional artists' rendition of this basically unattractive organ as the valentine. This pretty red figure bears little resemblance to the real item. The heart is the subject of countless poems, sonnets, and love songs, not to mention a bunch of clichés. We often use expressions such as "Follow your heart," or "Do what your heart tells you to do" when we advise someone who is struggling to make the right decision. Even those of us who understand very well the biological function of the heart talk as if our emotions are somehow connected to this fist-size pump!

Are we just being silly? No. It is not because of ignorance that the heart has become linked to feelings. During times of intense emotion, we have a heightened awareness of our heart. When we're scared, our hearts speed up. When we're extremely upset, we may feel a tightness in our chests, often experiencing the sensation of being "all choked up." When we suffer a severe disappointment, we may actually experience a sinking feeling that seems to emanate from our chests. And when we're madly in love, we may feel as if our hearts actually skip a beat when we encounter the object of our devotion. These sensations are real. They are caused by a series of biochemical reactions that enable the heart to adapt to stress. Thus, it is understandable that the earliest scientific thinkers bestowed such wondrous powers on this critical organ.

Although it wasn't until the middle of the twentieth century that we really began to understand the intricacies of the heart, some of its mysteries were unraveled by the medical researchers of antiquity. In A.D. 130, Galen, a personal physician to a Roman emperor, advanced the concept of a circulatory system through which blood flowed from the body to the heart and then back to the body. As chief physician to the gladiators, Galen presumably had many opportunities to study the inner workings of their bodies while tending to their wounds. (Even back then cardiac research was conducted principally on males!)

About a thousand years later, anatomists discovered that blood made an important detour through the lungs before being sent throughout the body. Some even suspected that blood was mixed with air in the lungs. Then, in 1517, British physician William Harvey put all the missing pieces together in his ground-breaking thesis *De Motu Cordis*. Harvey described the heart as a muscular chamber that functioned as a pump. In this brilliant essay, he also correctly described the circulatory system, showing that it was a closed circuit through which the blood travels through the heart, the lungs, and the rest of the body. Like many other great thinkers of his time, Harvey also equated the heart with man's soul and believed that it manufactured and imparted some "vital spirit" to the blood.

We now know that the heart is actually an elegantly designed organ that performs a vital service: It pumps life-sustaining blood to the rest of the body. Blood contains oxygen and nutrients necessary for the functioning of all the tissues and organs of the body—including the heart.

The heart is a muscular organ with four separate compartments, each of which performs a specific function. It consists of two upper chambers called atria and two lower chambers called ventricles. There are four special heart valves within the heart that open and snap shut to ensure that the blood flows in the right direction and doesn't back up into the chamber from which it has just come.

The heart is enclosed in a translucent sac called the pericardium. It is suspended in the chest from what are known as the great vessels: two muscular tubes called arteries. One of them, the pulmonary artery, carries blood to the lungs from the right-sided chambers of the heart, and the other, the aorta, distributes the freshly oxygenated blood to the rest of the body from the left-sided chambers. In most people, the heart is located on the left side of the upper portion of the chest. In some rare cases, however, a perfectly well-functioning heart may be found on the right side.

How blood flows to and from the healthy heart is outlined below. The diagram on page 6 is intended to help you visualize the process.

1. As we use blood, we take oxygen out of it and put carbon dioxide and waste materials into it. This "used" blood, which is dark bluish in color, flows through two large blood vessels—the superior vena cava and the inferior vena cava—into the right atrium of the heart.
2. After blood is collected in the right atrium, it passes through a passageway guarded by the tricuspid valve into the right ventricle. Then the right ventricle contracts. That contraction causes several things to happen. The contraction causes the tricuspid valve to shut so the blood doesn't flow backward into the right atrium. That same contraction also forces open the pulmonic valve. The pulmonic valve is the exit door. It opens into the pulmonary artery. The contraction forces blood through this exit door, into the pulmonary artery and then into the circulation of the lungs.
3. In the lungs, the blood gives up carbon dioxide and receives oxygen. The addition of oxygen turns blood a bright red. (The reason we think of blood as red is that when we see it, it *is* red, because it's on the outside of the body and is therefore exposed to oxygen.)

THE FEMALE HEART

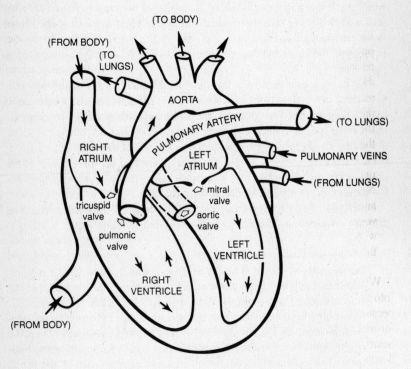

4. When the blood leaves the lungs, it passes through the pulmonary vein back to the left atrium of the heart.
5. After the blood is collected in the left atrium, it flows through the passageway guarded by the mitral valve into the left ventricle.
6. When it is filled with blood, the left ventricle contracts, pushing the blood into the great vessel we call the aorta. From the aorta, the blood flows to the rest of the body.
7. The blood, which is propelled through the body by the force of the left ventricular contraction, flows through vessels that gradually get smaller and smaller until the blood reaches the smallest vessels of all: the capillaries. In the capillaries another important exchange takes place, the opposite of what happens in the lungs. In the capillaries, oxygen is removed from the blood and delivered to our body tissues, and carbon dioxide and other waste products are removed from our tissues and put into the blood. Interestingly, one of the first organs to be fed is the heart itself. When blood is pumped out of the left ventricle into the arteries, the first arteries to receive it are the coronary arteries that branch off the aorta.
8. After the blood reaches the capillaries, where it delivers oxygen and picks up carbon dioxide and waste materials, it begins the trip back to the heart. Now blood flows from the capillaries into tiny veins and then into larger and larger vessels that eventually empty into the two vena cavae—the great veins that attach to the right atrium. This is where we began. Then the whole process is repeated again and again and again, never stopping, for the duration of our lives.

When the heart pumps blood into the aorta, the first place some of it goes is into the coronary arteries that feed the heart. This fact is important to know, because if anything obstructs the flow of blood through these coronary arteries for more than 30 minutes, the heart will not receive oxygen and parts of the heart muscle will be destroyed forever, which can mean disability or even death. That's why coronary artery disease, or CAD—a condition in which the coronary arteries become blocked or obstructed—is so dangerous.

If you put your hand over your heart, you will feel it beating—(contracting and relaxing)—about 60 times per minute, or 100,000 times per day. During a normal life span, a healthy heart will beat about 2.5 billion times. Its beating is regulated by a superbly coordinated sequence of electrical impulses that originate within the heart itself. Fortunately, the heart is programed to work automatically, no matter what other things we do, no matter whether we are conscious or unconscious, asleep or awake. And unlike most other muscles, the heart never really gets a chance to rest for any prolonged periods of time.

YOU'VE GOT RHYTHM

The heart muscle is actually a mass of two million living entities called *myocytes*, which literally means "muscle cells." Different kinds of cells perform different functions. The pumping action or beating of the heart is controlled by a specialized group of cells that produce a natural electrical impulse that causes the other cells to contract. The beat of a heart is a well-orchestrated event. It begins spontaneously in a special island of cells in the right atrium (the right upper chamber) called the sinus node. The sinus node is also referred to as the pacemaker of the heart. From the sinus node, that impulse is conducted in an orderly fashion by special conducting cells through the atrial muscle of both sides of the upper chambers of the heart. It then continues to the atrio-ventricular node, or the AV node, which lies in the floor of the right atrium. From the AV node, electrical waves are conducted to special conducting fibers that carry the pulse to all parts of the ventricles (the lower chambers). Since the electrical impulse penetrates the atria first, they contract a fraction of a second before the ventricles. This ensures their complete emptying and helps keep the leaflets of the tricuspid and mitral valves from ballooning backward into the upper chambers when the ventricles in turn contract.

If there is any disturbance in the normal sequence of the electrical impulse in either the rhythm of the beat that's generated or in the transmission of the impulse once it is formed, the result is a large category of disorders called arrhythmias. Although some arrhythmias are normal, certain kinds of arrhythmias can be deadly. In fact, as many as 400,000 Americans die from them each year (see chapter 7).

The electrical impulse, which triggers the contraction of the heart muscle, can actually be recorded on a device called an electrocardiograph, or EKG. Most of you have probably seen an EKG test result: It looks like a series of wavy lines drawn on a long piece of graph paper. But from these peaks and valleys, doctors are able to discern vital information about the heart, including whether or not a portion of the heart muscle has been injured due to lack of oxygen. Any disturbance or irregularity in the EKG may indicate a problem in the anatomy or function of the heart.

Although female and male hearts look exactly alike, it's interesting to note that their EKG tracings reveal different timing of a portion of the electrical complex. This difference between men and women appears only after puberty. No one knows why this is so, but hormones probably play a role.

THE FEMALE HEART: A SUM OF ITS PARTS

It wasn't until the middle of the twentieth century that researchers really began to understand fully the wonders of the heart and cardiovascular system. Part of this new appreciation of the heart comes from the work of cardiac researchers, myself included, who have studied the heart at the level of its individual molecules, rather than as a whole organ.

Most of my research has been at the cellular level. Each cell is a living entity encased in an outer membrane made up of lipids, proteins, and sugars. The heart is actually a community of approximately two billion specialized cells, tailored to help the heart perform its job.

There are three basic types of heart cells: (1) Atrial cells form the atria, or upper chambers; (2) ventricular myocardial cells form the ventricles; (3) and throughout the heart are specialized conducting cells that help transmit the electrical impulses that keep the heart beating. Every heart cell consists of three elements: (1) one or two nuclei, the part of the cell that contains genetic material; (2) little energy packets called mitochondria that provide fuel for work; and (3) contractile units called sarcomeres that enable the cells to shorten and relax again so that the heart can beat. The amount of each component varies according to how the cell is being used at the moment. Heart cells are not static: They are forever in flux. In fact, heart cells, like other muscle cells, can actually change their chemical composition to adapt to particular stresses.

Since the early 1970s, my colleagues and I have studied the way heart cells adapt to specific challenges. Based on our research, we have learned that from the time an infant takes her first breath to the moment when the heart beats for the very last time, the heart cells are constantly rearranging their molecular structure to accommodate new demands for work. It may sound more like science fiction than fact, but this information is critical.

Let's say a woman develops high blood pressure, a condition that occurs when muscle cells in the walls of branches of the arteries constrict, narrowing the blood vessels. When this happens, the heart must pump blood against a greater resistance in order to circulate it—as if trying to push gallons of water through a straw instead of a garden hose. Every time the left ventricle pushes blood through the aortic valve into the aorta, it must push harder than normal to counteract the increased resistance. In the short run, the woman's heart would react to this increased workload by creating more mitochondria, which are energy-producing units, to provide fuel for the effort. But shortly after this accommodation, the heart must learn to adapt another way. It begins to produce more sarcomeres, or contractile units, that have specially tailored proteins to help the heart develop tension more slowly but much more efficiently, so that it can meet the demand for increased work against the higher pressure without wasting energy.

But suppose this same heart is confronted with another challenge. Let's say this woman with high blood pressure decides to race up a flight of steps to catch a train. Her heart must suddenly start beating more rapidly to accommodate this new work demand. Her cells, adapted for slow and efficient beating, will not be able to cope with this challenge as well as the cells of a woman with normal blood pressure. If the demand for the more rapid rate is severe or prolonged enough, the heart could become overwhelmed—it might even stop beating.

Fortunately, most of the time, the heart can withstand an extraordinary amount of stress, thanks to the amazing ability of its cells to modify their structure and function to perform specific tasks. Every physical exertion doesn't result in a heart attack; every emotional shock isn't lethal. Portions of the heart muscle can die and other cells will take over. Parts of the heart can become injured and scarred, and the rest of the muscle will keep pumping away. Although the heart can take a tremendous amount of abuse, at some point the stresses can become too great and the heart may simply stop functioning. And as we have seen from the thwarted attempts of researchers who have tried to develop an artificial heart, the human heart is very difficult to duplicate. Thus, we must learn to care for the one we have.

THE DEVELOPING HEART

The hearts that we are born with are formed long before we ever take our first breath. The development of the heart into a four-chambered structure is completed during the first trimester of pregnancy. The heart begins as a simple tube that is fixed at either end and grows unevenly. The first major change in shape is the looping of the tube so that one part of it lies in front of the other. The second major change is the turning of the loop to the left; this is accompanied by the partitioning of the tube into four distinct chambers. Each pair of chambers is separated from the other by a valve. To produce a healthy, normal heart, these events must occur without a hitch. If the heart fails to loop or turn correctly, or if the chambers or valves don't develop properly, the baby may be born with congenital heart disease. Not all developmental defects are fatal or even serious. A lot depends on when the defect occurs, and how it will affect the overall functioning of the heart. (For some reason, women seem to be affected more by congenital heart disease than men, although no one knows why.)

In the uterus, the baby receives oxygen and nutrients from the mother via the placenta, an organ specifically grown to support the pregnancy. The balance of work in the uterus is done by the baby's right ventricle, which operates at much lower pressures than the heart will face after birth. At the moment of birth, when the lungs expand and the baby takes her first breath, the placenta is cut off as an option and the left ventricle must do a great deal more work than it did in utero. In a matter of seconds, the baby has to pump a greater volume of blood against a much higher pressure than she has been doing: The heart must adapt to its first great challenge. During the first three days of life, the connection between the aorta and the pulmonary artery, that exists in the womb, before the baby can use her lungs to breathe and supply oxygen to her blood, usually closes spontaneously. If it doesn't, it must be closed surgically.

New heart cells can only be produced during the first few weeks of life outside the womb. After that, unlike other organs such as the liver, the heart cannot regenerate itself. If heart cells are injured, they will not be replaced, although other heart cells may be able to compensate for their loss by enlarging or actually changing their structure.

I have devoted a great deal of my research to studying the cardiac changes that occur during development in the womb and the first precious days and months of life. This brief period of time is of interest to researchers because many of the challenges that the normal infant's heart must face are similar to challenges that may occur later in life. For instance, the way the left ventricle adapts to a sudden increase in blood pressure immediately after birth has shed important light on ways in which the adult heart adapts to a sudden increase in pressure. In understanding how the heart adapts to normal stress during the growth and development of the child, we have learned a great deal about how the adult heart meets and deals with demands for increased work.

This all-important early stage of life may teach us other crucially important lessons. For example, if we can figure out why the baby can produce new heart cells—an ability that suddenly stops by the third week of life—we may be able to somehow extend this period so we can develop a reserve of healthy heart cells that can be used if other cardiac cells are destroyed due to disease. We might even be able to reactivate the ability to make new cells in adults if we understand the conditions in newborns that make it possible to do so!

I think it's important to remember, however, that finding medical solutions to cardiac problems is only a second-best approach. It is far better to prevent the onset of disease in the first place. Most of us are born with clear arteries, clean lungs, and a healthy, strong heart. Heart disease is not an inevitable part of the aging process: It is often the result of neglect and abuse of our bodies. Very often, changes in lifestyle can reap terrific dividends in terms of health and well-being.

II

WHY WOMEN
ARE DIFFERENT

❧

Chapter 2

ANATOMY
OF A WOMAN

CORONARY artery disease has been the number one killer of both men and women since 1910. However, there are important differences in both the anatomy and lifestyle of women that profoundly affect susceptibility to heart disease, and the course the disease takes.

The first and most obvious difference is body size: Women tend to be smaller than men. As a result, most everything else in our bodies is scaled down accordingly. Not only is the typical female heart smaller than the male heart but the coronary arteries—the vessels that supply blood and oxygen to the heart—are also smaller and narrower. Due to their smaller size, it may take less plaque to block a coronary artery in a woman and impair the flow of blood and oxygen to her heart. There are studies to suggest that women's coronary arteries may also contract or narrow more vigorously than men's in response to the same stress. If all things were equal, women would get heart attacks earlier than men, but just the opposite is true. Although CAD is the leading cause of death in men age thirty-nine and older, it does not become the leading cause of death in women until age sixty. In fact, between ages forty and forty-nine, men are seven times more likely to develop CAD than women of the same age. What protects younger women, but not younger men, against the ravages of CAD? Sex hormones that regulate the menstrual cycle—specifically estrogen—are believed to offer women special protection against heart disease. However, once a woman becomes menopausal and her production of estrogen begins to taper off, her risk for developing CAD steadily climbs each year. At any age, women who experience premature menopause or undergo a premenopausal hysterectomy have a *threefold risk increase* for CAD for the rest of their lives!

When CAD finally strikes women, it hits hard and fast. If the heart is denied sufficient oxygen for about 30 minutes, the result will be a heart attack—that is, death of a portion of the heart tissue. In many ways, a heart attack is a far more serious event for a woman than it is for a man. When a

15

woman has a heart attack, she is twice as likely as a man to die within the first 60 days. In fact, 39 percent of all women heart attack victims will die within the first year of the attack versus 31 percent of all men. After that, she is twice as likely to have a second heart attack as a man. At any age, a woman is at greater risk of dying of a heart attack than a man. A major Israeli study involving 4,315 men and 1,524 women who had heart attacks between 1981 and 1983 revealed that even when women were compared with men of the same age, they experienced a strikingly higher mortality rate. According to this study, women suffered a 23 percent death rate during their initial hospital stay versus only 10 percent for men of the same age. For those who survived the heart attack, the one-year mortality rate was 12 percent as compared to only 9 percent for men of the same age.

Not only is a heart attack more lethal for women than for men but treatments for CAD are not as effective. Coronary artery bypass surgery—a procedure in which surgeons take a blood vessel from another part of the body and use it to construct a detour around the blocked portion of the coronary artery—is not as successful for women as it is for men; neither is balloon angioplasty, a procedure in which a deflated balloon on a catheter is passed through the artery and then inflated to open the obstruction and flatten the plaque against the artery wall. The road to recovery after surgery is also rockier for women, who are more likely to complain of depression, sexual dysfunction, and side effects from medications.

The later age at which heart attack strikes women may be partially responsible for the overall higher rate of death and other complications. The older you are, the harder it is for you—physically and psychically—to mend after a traumatic event such as a heart attack. You are also more likely to be widowed or living alone, which means that you may not be receiving proper care or emotional support at home after surgery. Female anatomy may also affect the outcome of surgery: The fact that female hearts and arteries are smaller may make it more difficult for the cardiac surgeon to perform angioplasty or a coronary bypass. The smaller female body size may also play a role in the fact that the standard dose for cardiac medication may be too high for women, thus explaining the reported increase in side effects.

SEX BIAS IN DIAGNOSIS OF FEMALE HEART DISEASE

Neither age, body size, nor marital status fully explain why women cardiac patients fare so poorly compared to men. The real reason may stem from the fact that women cardiac patients may be sicker than men to begin with, because they are diagnosed and treated at a later stage in the disease. In many cases, women or their doctors—or both—have ignored or neglected important warning signs. I believe that if these women are diagnosed and treated promptly, their prognosis is vastly improved. A case in point is a recent study done at the Cedars-Sinai Medical Center in Los Angeles. The study monitored 1,815 men and 482 women bypass patients between 1982 and 1987. The researchers suggested that there was a definite bias against referring women for bypass surgery: In order for a woman to be operated on, she had to be significantly sicker than a man. The researchers felt that the advanced state of the disease—not necessarily age—was the main reason why twice as many women in their study died from the surgery than men (4.6 percent female patients died versus 2.6 percent male patients). The study also suggested that doctors were not referring women for diagnostic testing in a timely fashion, ignoring symptoms in women that they would have probably acted upon in men.

The Cedars-Sinai findings confirmed a 1987 study done at the Albert Einstein College of Medicine in New York that suggested there was a sex bias in referring women for cardiac catheterization and angiography, the "gold standard" for diagnosing CAD. During cardiac catheterization, a thin tube or catheter is passed through a vein or artery into the heart. The tube is guided into each of the coronary arteries in turn and dye is injected into the vessel. Catheterization is used to determine the extent and course of CAD and to see if bypass surgery or angioplasty would be beneficial. The researchers reviewed the records of 390 patients referred for a thallium exercise stress test—137 women and 253 men—and found that 31 percent of the women and 64 percent of the men had abnormal results; 40 percent of the men with abnormal results were referred for cardiac catheterization. However, out of the group of women with abnormal test results, only 4 percent were referred for catheterization. In 84.3 percent of the males who tested abnormal, their cardiologists attributed their symptoms to a cardiac problem, but only 67.2 percent of the women were believed to have cardiac problems. What's even more interesting is that the cardiologists found that only 3 percent of the men had symptoms related to psychiatric problems, as compared to a whopping 10.9 percent of the women!

The Einstein and the Cedars-Sinai studies are particularly shocking because if they are indicative of other medical facilities—and they probably are—then many women may be suffering and even dying unnecessarily. I believe that these findings may reflect a tendency among many physicians to dismiss women's complaints as trivial and unimportant. Often, when a woman complains, she is stereotyped as a "whining, hysterical female"—a "head case." But when a man complains, it is automatically assumed that since men are usually more "stoic" about pain than women, he must really be in trouble. The study may also reflect ignorance on the part of many physicians who are so convinced that women don't get CAD that they don't even consider the possibility; therefore, they neglect to investigate important symptoms.

What I find even more upsetting is that these studies confirm my own personal observation that women are not as assertive as they should be on their own behalf. Most women who get heart attacks have experienced intermittent bouts of chest pain or angina long before the actual attack. In many cases, I believe if these women had received proper treatment for their problem—in some cases, medication or surgery—and made necessary changes in their lifestyle, they may have been able to avert the heart attack altogether, or at least, lessened its severity. However, I suspect that many of these women may have too easily accepted their doctor's assurances that they had nothing to worry about, or may even have neglected to report the chest pain to their doctors in the first place.

In defense of doctors, I want to add that women do experience chest pain more often than men and that it is not always caused by CAD. For instance, about 7 percent of all women have a usually benign congenital defect called mitral valve prolapse that can cause pain that can sometimes be confused with angina. In addition, women are more prone to develop spasm of the coronary arteries, which means that for some unknown reason a perfectly clear artery can suddenly constrict or narrow, reducing the flow of blood to the heart. However, there is no way of determining the cause of chest pain unless a woman is thoroughly examined by her physician.

Any chest pain should be investigated for the possibility of CAD whether the patient is male or female. At a very minimum, the physician should perform an electrocardiogram (EKG) to look for signs of damage to the heart muscle or arrhythmia. She should also perform an echocardiogram, a noninvasive test that uses sound waves to examine the structure and function of the heart muscle. In some cases, an exercise stress test may be useful to look for evidence of ischemia or oxygen deprivation, or the patient may be asked to wear a Holter monitor (a small computer which records part of the electrocardiogram periodically over a 24-hour period) to detect periods of ischemia (periods of time in which the blood supply to the heart is insufficient to maintain it). Unless your doctor has made a serious effort to discover the cause of your chest pain, you should not accept her assurances that you are okay.

Under the best of circumstances, it is often more difficult to diagnose CAD in women than in men. Not only are symptoms such as chest pain more confusing but the standard diagnostic tests are often not as accurate for women. For example, in about 10 percent of all cases, the standard exercise stress test will show CAD in people who don't have it, typically misdiagnosing women more than men. Even the highly accurate thallium stress test, which uses a radioactive substance to trace the flow of blood through the heart, is trickier to perform on women because breast tissue can obstruct the view of the heart. Physicians have to be especially alert in identifying women who are at high risk for CAD among their patients and must follow these women closely for any symptoms that could suggest CAD.

It's not just doctors who are ignoring important symptoms on the part of their female patients. Often, the patients are just as responsible. In fact, studies show that many women may neglect to call their doctors even when they are having a full-blown heart attack. About 35 percent of all heart attacks in women (as opposed to only 27 percent in men) go unnoticed because the victim either believes the pain is angina or some noncardiac problem such as indigestion. Sometimes, in the case of the so-called "silent heart attack," there may be no pain at all. I believe, however, the fact that more than one-third of all women's heart attacks go unreported also reflects denial on the part of many women who simply prefer to believe that the pain was only a minor malady. When the pain goes away, the heart attack victim is only too happy to assume that everything is all right and she often forgets about the incident. At some later date an irregular EKG will reveal the scarring or damage left by a previous heart attack.

THE ROLE OF SEX HORMONES IN A WOMAN'S LIFE

The physical differences between men and women extend far beyond cardiology. Because women produce an ovum every month, their bodies are sensitive to monthly fluctuations in hormones that regulate the menstrual cycle. As I said earlier in this chapter, female sex hormones seem to play a major role in protecting women against CAD. But once hormone production falls after menopause, that protection soon disappears. In order to fully understand the role hormones play in preventing heart disease, you must first understand the critical role hormones play in every woman's life.

Hormones are chemicals produced by a collection of glands and other organs called the endocrine system. Specific hormones have specific jobs. Hormones released by the adrenal glands trigger the body's reaction to stress: the so-called "fight or flight" response. Other hormones regulate digestion and help the body break down nutrients from food. Still other hormones regulate sexual development and growth. The heart itself secretes a hormone called atrial natriuretic factor that is believed to help regulate blood pressure.

Within the past few decades, we have gained much understanding about how hormones work. As a result, we are now able to produce synthetic hormones that work in much the same way as the real thing. Today, millions of women take synthetic hormones for a variety of reasons. Some use them to promote fertility.

Others take birth control pills. And still others rely on them to alleviate the discomfort of menopause. Some experts have even suggested that since a drop in estrogen seems to increase the risk of heart disease, women should routinely take synthetic estrogen as a precaution against CAD. But before we can decide whether it's a good idea to take synthetic estrogen after menopause, let's examine the role of natural sex hormones produced by our bodies.

Let's begin at the point where life begins. There are four stages in the process of becoming a woman that shape our physical and psychological development. The first stage begins at the moment of conception. When a woman's egg unites with a man's sperm, each contributes 23 single chromosomes to create a new cell with a total of 46 chromosomes. Chromosomes are tiny, rodlike structures inside the nucleus of every body cell. Each chromosome consists of thousands of genes, which are chemicals that store information. There are about 100,000 genes in total, and each one determines a different trait or characteristic.

Within these chromosomes lie the blueprint for the new life. At the moment of fertilization, the child's sex is determined by the father, who donates either an X or a Y chromosome to match the mother's X chromosome. If the child is XX, it is a girl. If it is XY, it is a boy.

The second stage occurs in males during the sixth to eighth week of life in the womb, and in females at around the ninth week. During this period, the reproductive glands or gonads begin to form. Boys develop testes. Girls grow ovaries. The gonads secrete specific hormones that trigger further sexual development. The testes produce testosterone and the ovaries produce estrogen. Testosterone is associated with so-called "masculine" attributes such as the growth of body hair, the development of muscles, and overall aggressive behavior. Women also produce testosterone, but in much lower levels than men. The presence, or lack, of testosterone is critical for the third stage: the growth of external genitals. Testosterone will stimulate the development of a penis. Without testosterone, the embryo will develop a vagina.

The three major stages of sexual development—genetic, gonadal, and genital—are completed by the third month of gestation. But the fourth stage of becoming a woman—of developing a distinctly female identity—begins immediately after birth. Regardless of genetics, sexual identity—the psychological aspects of sexuality that determine how we feel and how we behave— are significantly affected by how we are reared. In fact, if a child is treated as a female from birth, she will be a female psychologically for the rest of her life, whether or not Mother Nature intended her to be one.

The sexual and psychological identity of a female is completed within the first 24 months of life. The groundwork has been laid for the physical and emotional development of a woman. After this critical period, a female's biological clock takes over, following a blueprint established back in the womb.

PUBERTY: BECOMING A WOMAN, BECOMING PROTECTED FROM CAD

For many people, just the mention of the word *puberty* conjures up some very uncomfortable memories: pimples, training bras, first dates, sweaty palms, inexplicable mood swings. Despite all the outer awkwardness, inside her body the hormones are doing their job with exquisite precision. Sometime, usually between her twelfth or thirteenth birthday, a girl enters into puberty, or experiences her first menstrual cycle. When a girl is born, she is endowed with a million eggs in her ovaries. By the time she reaches adolescence, the number is halved. But when she reaches the age of menstruation, about 50 of these eggs begin to ripen each month in preparation for fertilization.

The menstrual cycle is caused by the activation of certain key hormones that prepare a woman's body for pregnancy. It all begins in the brain. The hypothalamus puts out gonadotropin-releasing hormones (GNRH). GNRH directs the pituitary, the body's master gland, to produce follicle-stimulating hormones (FSH). FSH stimulates the production of a follicle within the ovary. Luteinizing hormones (LH) stimulate the ovaries to produce estrogen. At around 14 days, or midcycle, the ripened egg or ovum is released to begin its journey down the fallopian tube. The corpus luteum, the follicle shed by the egg, remains in the ovary and begins to secrete both estrogen and another hormone, progesterone. During the first half of the menstrual cycle, estrogen helps to build up the uterine lining, or endometrium, so it will be able to nourish the fertilized egg after implantation. During the second half, or progesterone phase, of the cycle, progesterone finishes the job by further preparing the endometrium to receive the ovum. If the egg isn't fertilized and pregnancy doesn't occur, progesterone shifts gears and helps break down the uterine lining so it can be shed during menstruation.

A girl's body undergoes other miraculous changes during this rite of passage. Prior to the onset of puberty, girls typically experience their last growth spurt. They often shoot up before filling out, frequently towering over their male classmates. Boys catch up a year or two later. Once puberty begins, however, estrogen prevents the bone cells from dividing as rapidly as before, thus diminishing future growth. Subcutaneous fat is deposited under the skin: Angles now become curves; a woman's skin stays soft and supple. Breasts begin to grow and develop. For some mysterious reason, both boys and girls experience a drop in cholesterol levels right before puberty begins, probably due to increased hormonal levels. The reproductive system continues to gear up for motherhood as the uterine muscles and lining both grow. The vaginal mucus thickens and increases in acid content in preparation for future intercourse.

Over a 30-year period, the average woman will experience approximately

400 menstrual cycles, minus a year or two, depending on the number of times she is pregnant. By her mid-forties, her body readies itself to embark on another major life change: menopause.

MENOPAUSE: THE COMING OF AGE AND INCREASED RISK FOR CAD

Menopause, sometimes called the change of life, is another rite of passage that ushers in a new phase of female growth and development. Once again, a shift in hormonal levels triggers major bodily changes. During the ages of forty-five to fifty-five, most women begin to notice a change in their monthly menstrual cycle. Although the average age for the onset of menopause is between forty-five and fifty-five, around 8 percent of all women have early, spontaneous menopause before age forty. No one knows why some women have it earlier than others, but we suspect genetics plays a role. If your mother had an early menopause, chances are that you will too.

As the number of available eggs in the ovaries begins to dwindle, ovulation becomes less frequent. The ovaries, in turn, begin to produce less estrogen, probably because there is no longer any reason to build up the uterine lining in preparation for pregnancy. Periods become erratic, lighter, and slowly begin to taper off. It could be several years before menstruation ceases entirely. Although we use the term *menopause* to describe an entire stage of life, the word actually refers to the last menstrual period. Once menstruation stops, the ovaries still produce estrogen, but at a much lower level than before.

A word of caution: If you stop bleeding for any six-month period, and then suddenly resume bleeding, check immediately with your doctor. This is not a normal sign of menopause and could indicate any number of problems—some serious, some not. Don't play guessing games. Make an appointment to see your physician.

After menopause, a woman's natural protection against developing CAD disappears. By her sixty-fifth birthday, she is at equal risk with men for heart attack and is even more likely to develop high blood pressure. In addition, once a woman stops menstruating, her low-density lipoprotein (LDL) level rises and her level of high-density lipoprotein (HDL)—the good cholesterol—drops. The increase in LDL is believed to be directly related to the drop in estrogen production by the ovaries.

As estrogen levels dip, the body begins to experience other changes. The uterus and vagina start to shrink; the vaginal lining and urethral lining begin to thin, making a woman more vulnerable to urinary and vaginal infections. The vagina produces less lubricant, and when this factor is combined with the thinner vaginal lining, intercourse may be painful. The layer of fat under the skin begins to shrink, making the skin less soft and supple. While pubic and leg hair may decrease, facial hair may appear on many women.

At this stage in life, many women begin to develop osteoporosis, or bone loss. It is believed that the reduction in estrogen interferes with the body's ability to absorb dietary calcium, an essential ingredient in bone production. As a result, the big bones become brittle and more prone to fractures and breaks.

During the period leading up to and immediately following menopause, some women experience other disturbing symptoms including headaches, excessive fatigue, dizziness, insomnia, arrhythmia, palpitations, and even depression. The infamous hot flashes are probably one of the most uncomfortable aspects of menopause. Although some women never get them, many menopausal women are made miserable by them. A typical hot flash is a sudden feeling of intense heat, accompanied by heavy sweating and extreme discomfort. It may last for several minutes. Hot flashes are caused by increased production of FSH and LH by the pituitary in a frantic effort to stimulate ovulation. Despite this barrage of hormones, the ovaries usually lie fallow. (Of course, there are exceptions. We've all heard of "change of life" babies. That's why women are advised to use contraception until one full year after their last menstrual cycle.) The hormonal imbalance caused by the release of these hormones somehow interferes with the body's normal heat-regulating systems. Your doctor may refer to this condition as a disturbance of the vasomotor system. Some women may have a few mild hot flashes throughout the day, whereas others may be bombarded with one intense hot flash after another, especially at night. Fortunately, hot flashes usually disappear within a year or two after your body adjusts to the hormonal changes of menopause. But for some women, it can be a time of sheer agony.

Women who are heavy smokers tend to have menopause between five and ten years earlier than women who don't smoke. Even light smokers may become menopausal up to three years earlier than they might if they didn't smoke.

Menopause affects women differently. Some women hardly notice any symptoms, whereas others can't help but notice the minute-to-minute bodily changes that are wreaking havoc on their lives. Although no one knows why some women are affected more than others, it's possible that estrogen production may fall off gradually in some lucky women, creating milder symptoms. Others may suddenly have to deal with the equivalent of a hormonal roller-coaster ride. Psychological factors may also be at play here. I have treated women who equate the loss of ovarian function with the loss of femininity and the beginning of a "neutered," old age. Many mourn menopause as though it was the end of life itself, and for these women, the adjustment is especially difficult.

Although there are some women who may mourn the end of their child-bearing years, I believe that there are just as many women who are delighted to say goodbye to premenstrual syndrome (PMS), menstrual cramps, and monthly periods. And yes, there are even some who are thrilled at the prospect of being able to indulge in sex without having to give a second thought of becoming pregnant. However, even if you embrace menopause with open arms, you may still experience some discomfort as your body adjusts to the hormonal fluctuations.

HYSTERECTOMY OR SURGICALLY INDUCED MENOPAUSE AND EARLY RISK FOR HEART DISEASE

Hysterectomy, the surgical removal of all or part of the uterus, is the second most commonly performed operation in the United States (only cesarean sections are performed more often). It is often accompanied by removal of one or both of the ovaries in a procedure called salpingo-oophorectomy. If a woman loses her uterus and ovaries, she will become menopausal and her risk for developing CAD dramatically increases.

At 800,000 per year, there are more hysterectomies performed in the United States than in any other country in the world. In fact, if present trends continue, 62 percent of all adult women today will have a hysterectomy sometime during their lives. There has been much controversy over these figures. Consumer groups and even many doctors contend that as many as 50 percent of all hysterectomies are unnecessary, performed by surgeons who may be thinking more of their pocketbooks than of their patients. Indeed, studies have shown that the rate of hysterectomy is significantly higher in areas such as the Southwest where there is a greater concentration of surgeons. Opponents of hysterectomy feel that the operation is often performed for the wrong reasons, and often alternative therapies are ignored. For instance, these critics contend that many women with mild fibroid tumors or benign uterine bleeding need not lose their uterus, although these are two of the most common reasons the surgery is performed.

Some women feel the emotional aftershocks of hysterectomy long after the physical wounds have healed. Many complain of depression, loss of libido, and painful intercourse. Having a hysterectomy can be very traumatic; nevertheless, there are times when it is absolutely necessary. For example, for women who have uterine cancer it can be a true lifesaver. There are also times when hysterectomy may not be necessary to save a woman's life, but it can vastly improve her quality of life. For instance, if she suffers from a severely or displaced prolapsed uterus—her uterus has dropped down into her vagina—she may benefit from surgery.

There are times, however, when hysterectomy may do more harm than good. According to recent studies, women who undergo premenopausal hysterectomies have a threefold increase of CAD for the rest of their lives. In fact, researchers in one study group bluntly said that to be absolutely certain that "premenopausal hysterectomies do not cause more deaths due to cardio-vascular disease than they save by preventing uterine cancer requires a per-spective study of 20,000 women observed until death." In other words, more studies are needed to assess the true risk versus the benefits of premenopausal hysterectomy. Women must carefully weigh the facts before undergoing such surgery. Ask your doctor about alternatives to surgery. If your case is not acute, she may be able to try other treatments before resorting to surgery. In some communities, medical consumer groups can provide additional information on other options, such as the National Women's Health Network in Washington, D.C.

I firmly believe that if you're faced with the prospect of premenopausal hysterectomy, you must consider the effect it will have on increasing your risk of heart disease. Therefore, I carefully review with my patient's gynecologist a decision to do a hysterectomy. I sometimes advise a woman who has been told that she needs a hysterectomy to get a second opinion. In many cases, thanks to new surgical techniques, conditions that were once believed to require hysterectomy, such as small uterine fibroid tumors, can be removed without endangering the uterus, or even treated with medication.

You and your doctor must review your family history of heart disease and hypertension, as well as consider your own risk factors. You must weigh these risk factors against your chances of developing a life-threatening disease such as cancer, or spending the rest of your life in pain due to a uterine problem. With the help of your doctor, you should be able to make an informed decision.

Chapter 3

SYNTHETIC HORMONES
AND THE HEART

FOR years, the changing hormone levels associated with menopause have been suspected of contributing to the sudden rise of heart disease in women. Since the mid-1980s, we have begun to come up with some answers. Although we don't have the whole story, we do have enough information to piece together some of the puzzle.

After puberty, women typically have higher levels of high-density lipoproteins (HDL), the "good" cholesterol, and lower levels of low-density lipoproteins (LDL), the "bad" cholesterol, than do men. But once a woman stops menstruating, her HDL drops, her LDL rises, and her overall cholesterol level increases. Nearly everyone agrees that the decline in estrogen production by the ovaries is a major contributor to the change in blood lipids.

What does estrogen—a sex hormone—have to do with HDL and LDL? According to a recent study in the *New England Journal of Medicine*, estrogen plays a major role in the way lipids are produced, handled, broken down, and even eliminated from the body. In this study, postmenopausal women were given synthetic estrogen supplements, known as estrogen replacement therapy, or ERT. Women on ERT had a reduction in LDL, which is good, and a dramatic rise in HDL, which is even better. There was one negative side effect: Taking ERT resulted in a moderate increase in triglycerides. Elevated triglycerides are a significant risk factor in women for developing heart disease. Why did these three things happen? The researchers proposed that the synthetic estrogen might somehow promote a change in the shape or electrical charge of HDL particles, making them able to carry fewer triglycerides, so that blood triglyceride levels rose.

Since estrogen has a mostly positive effect on blood lipids, some medical experts believe that the hormone should be taken after natural menopause or premenopausal hysterectomy to compensate for the loss of ovarian function. Indeed, whether or not routinely to prescribe ERT to all postmenopausal women in order to prevent heart disease is a burning question in the medical community today. Millions of women are already taking ERT to help alleviate some of the more unpleasant symptoms of menopause, such as hot flashes and thinning of the vaginal wall, which can cause pain during sexual intercourse.

Some women take ERT for short periods of time until their body adjusts to menopause, whereas others require long-term treatment. Women at high risk of osteoporosis, bone destruction, or shrinkage due to calcium deficiency are often given ERT to prevent the onset of this potentially debilitating disease or to prevent further bone loss, although there is no evidence that it prevents fractures. What has proven to be of most interest to internists and cardiologists, however, is that a handful of studies also confirm that women on ERT have a 30 percent to 50 percent reduction in the development of CAD compared with menopausal women not taking any replacement therapy.

The widespread use of ERT has generated much controversy—especially among women's health groups—for several reasons. First, critics claim that there have not been enough studies to demonstrate that ERT is safe for long-term use. As of yet, there are no long-range studies following ERT patients from menopause through old age. Second, some of the existing studies do not give ERT a clean bill of health. In fact, they have demonstrated a connection between the use of ERT and the development of uterine cancer. Certain kinds of estrogen-sensitive breast cancer too small for detection may be stimulated to grow by ERT. Finally, these critics object to ERT on philosophical grounds. They bristle at the notion that menopause is an "illness" that requires drug intervention. In fact, some say that ERT is being pushed on unsuspecting women—who neither need it nor want it—by drug companies interested in making profits.

On the other side, ERT's proponents—endocrinologists, many gynecologists, and many women who take the drug—often make it sound as if it is a veritable fountain of youth. In fact, one popular book on the subject claims that ERT promotes "great sex, strong bones, good looks, longer life," in addition to preventing hot flashes!

This controversy has been widely reported in the popular press. Nearly every woman who comes to my office has read a newspaper or a magazine article touting this amazing treatment that not only makes you feel and look younger and sexier but guards against heart disease too. Chances are, though, that these same women have seen other articles describing studies that cast doubt on the safety of ERT.

Where do I stand in this controversy? Right where I think every good doctor should stand: firmly in the middle. Every patient is different—no one treatment should be uniformly prescribed for everyone. Before a doctor writes a prescription for ERT or any other medication, each woman should be evaluated on an individual basis, and the risks and benefits should be clearly spelled out for the patient. In situations such as ERT where treatment is usually optional, I work with the patient to help her reach a decision. Equally important, once the medication is prescribed, I watch my patient very carefully, especially those who must take progesterone along with the estrogen. For example, a small percentage of women on ERT (less than 10 percent) experience mood swings, become intensely anxious, and even become depressed—symptoms similar to premenstrual syndrome (PMS). While this reaction is unusual, and was more common when higher doses of estrogen were used than are usually used today, it is still a valid reason for not using the drug.

There is no question, however, that for some women ERT is a godsend, especially for those with a strong family history of osteoporosis. Hormonal intervention may save these women from developing fragile bones and from experiencing the subsequent breaks and injuries that often result in confinement to a wheelchair or life in a nursing home. For other women, however, I believe ERT's benefits are mainly psychological. Many mourn menopause as though it were the end of life itself and regard ERT as an antidote to death and aging. More than one of my patients claim that without their daily dose of estrogen, their skin would shrivel up, their energy level would plummet, and their sex life would become nonexistent. Frankly, I question whether their life would be that dismal without their daily estrogen fix. But despite my skepticism, I'm glad that estrogen works for these women and would not dream of taking their hormones away without a pretty compelling reason.

ERT is usually not prescribed until menstruation ceases, but in very rare cases it may be given if a woman has experienced severe symptoms while entering a full-blown menopause. ERT can be administered in several ways:

1. *Oral preparation:* Premarin, the brand name for the most commonly prescribed oral estrogen, is metabolized or broken down by the liver before it is absorbed by the bloodstream.
2. *Estrogen cream:* In the form of a cream, estrogen can be used to reduce irritation caused by the thinning vaginal tissue. Inserted into the vagina via an applicator, the estrogen does not circulate through the liver and is absorbed directly into the blood.
3. *Transdermal patch:* Estrogen can also be delivered to the body via a Band-Aid-like patch worn low on the abdomen or buttocks. Estrogen given by this route bypasses the liver and is absorbed directly through the skin. It is marketed under the name Estraderm. The patch delivers a steady stream of .05 mg (or 0.1 mg) of estrogen and must be changed twice a week.

ERT AND CANCER

Early ERT studies showed an increased risk of uterine cancer due to the buildup of the endometrium or uterine lining in women who still had a uterus. (During menstruation, estrogen stimulates endometrium to prepare the uterus to receive the fertilized egg.) To solve this problem, progestin, a synthetic form of progesterone, was given in addition to the estrogen to perform the role it plays in the monthly menstrual cycle: to break down the uterine lining so it can be discharged through the vagina. The most common form of progestin used today is Provera. Women on combination estrogen/progestin therapy usually take progestin for ten to thirteen days each month. Most women have short menstrual-like periods immediately following the progestin regime. The periods usually disappear within a few years after menopause when the endometrium ceases to function.

With the addition of progestin, the risk of uterine cancer declined, but it was replaced by a new and more deadly risk: breast cancer. A group of researchers in Sweden who followed 23,000 women on estrogen/progestin therapy found that the rate of breast cancer was four times higher in women on hormones than in women who didn't take any. This came as no surprise to some doctors who had been warning all along that progestin can stimulate growth of breast tissue. Proponents of ERT, however, have been quick to point out that the estrogen compound used in Sweden is different than that used in the United States.

It is also important to point out that the growth of some types of breast cancer is enhanced by estrogen; if a woman has a previously undetected and estrogen-sensitive tumor of the breast, and begins to take hormone therapy, her cancer will grow faster than if she were not taking estrogen. I feel that it's unclear whether the progestin contributes to the growth of cancerous tumors, or whether estrogen itself stimulates the growth of an existing tumor. Even if ERT may slightly increase the risk of breast cancer, it still does not negate the positive effects of estrogen, especially on blood lipids. As ERT's proponents remind us, ten times as many women die each year of heart disease as those with breast cancer.

What is probably more important to consider is the effect of progestin on the positive results of taking estrogen. Although estrogen has been shown to have beneficial effects on blood lipid levels, progestin has just the opposite effect. In fact, certain types of potent progestins actually counteract estrogen by causing HDL to drop and LDL to rise.

ERT AND CAD

There are still many unanswered questions about ERT. There are a few studies—albeit a minority—that fail to demonstrate any reduction in CAD for women on ERT. Interestingly enough, the Framingham study did not show that ERT reduced the incidence of CAD among postmenopausal women taking the replacement therapy. In fact, women who used postmenopausal estrogen were at more than a 50 percent higher risk for stroke. In smokers who used estrogen, there were higher rates of heart attacks than in other women. It is not known whether estrogen taken via the transdermal or skin patch will have any positive effect on blood lipids since it is not metabolized by the liver; this question has never been properly studied. Finally, we simply don't know whether progestin poses more potential risks to cardiovascular health than it is worth.

Some of these questions may be answered by a study currently underway by the National Heart, Lung and Blood Institute. The Post Menopausal Estrogen/Progestin Intervention Trials, or PEPI Trials, began in October 1989. The study will examine the effect of various estrogen/progestin treatments, including the patch, on women between the ages of forty-five and sixty-four. The study will also monitor the effect of these hormones on blood lipids and will watch the participants closely to see if they show a reduction in cardiovascular disease, or an increase in cancer. Short-term results should be available within the next five years, but it will be decades before we know the long-term effects of this treatment.

Some women will prefer to pass on ERT until all the data are in. Ultimately, the decision to take ERT is up to the individual woman and her physician. Although I can't tell you whether or not ERT will work for you, I can tell you how I decide which patients, in my opinion, should steer clear of estrogen therapy. Although some doctors dismiss the progestin/breast cancer link, I do not. Thus, I feel very strongly that every woman should have a mammogram before embarking on this treatment to detect any hidden breast tumors that could be aggravated by either estrogen or progestin. The mammogram should be repeated each year.

Second, if a woman on ERT has a close relative—mother, grandmother, sister—who has had breast cancer, an annual mammogram is not enough. Every six months, she should be examined by a breast cancer specialist. I would not recommend ERT in any form to any woman who has had a history of blood clots, smokes, or is hypertensive (estrogen can raise blood pressure). Since estrogen raises triglyceride levels, I would not give this medication to any woman who already has a history of elevated triglycerides. Finally, I would be reluctant to prescribe ERT to any woman who has had a history of depression. If I did give it to her, I would monitor her very closely for signs of a recurrence.

We don't yet know enough about this treatment to prescribe it on a routine basis to women purely as a means of preventing heart disease. I would feel perfectly comfortable prescribing ERT to a healthy woman, without any of the previously cited risk factors, who has had a hysterectomy and is suffering the effects of estrogen deprivation. This woman can take estrogen in its pure form, undiluted by progestin. I would also give ERT to a woman without other risk factors, who is most likely to develop osteoporosis, or already shows signs of this debilitating bone disease. Those at greatest risk are women of Caucasian or Asian descent who are slender and small-boned. Women who smoke, drink excessively, have sedentary lifestyles, and fail to get adequate calcium in their diets are also at high risk.

If a woman is experiencing severe symptoms of menopause and can't find any relief from other remedies, ERT may be helpful. For example, if a woman's ability to enjoy sex is being impaired by painful intercourse, and over-the-counter personal lubricants are ineffective, I would gladly write a prescription for estrogen cream. If it didn't work, I would even suggest a transdermal patch. I believe that good health goes hand in hand with emotional well-being.

Any woman on ERT must be closely monitored by her physician, and must carefully be checked for endometrial cancer at least every six months. In some cases, the doctor may do an endometrial biopsy, a procedure in which uterine cells are suctioned through the cervix and examined for hyperplasia, or abnormal cell growth. Although this procedure is usually not very painful—the cervix is not dilated—it can cause some discomfort. After age fifty, annual mammograms are a must, for all women, but especially for those on hormones.

ORAL CONTRACEPTIVES: HIGH BLOOD PRESSURE AND CARDIOVASCULAR DISEASE

There are some very compelling reasons why approximately ten million American women take the pill. It is easy to use, it improves spontaneity in sexual relations, and most important, it prevents unwanted pregnancy in 97 percent to 99 percent of its users. There are also some good reasons why many women should not take birth control pills. Although oral contraceptives are a very efficient means of preventing pregnancy, they are not without risk. As a

RESOURCES: See page 233.

cardiologist, I am most concerned about the significant numbers of women on oral contraceptives who develop high blood pressure. According to one comprehensive study, about 5 percent of women on the pill will develop hypertension—blood pressures of 140/90 or higher—within a five-year period. This statistic is more than double the normal risk of becoming hypertensive. The likelihood of developing high blood pressure increases if you are overweight, over thirty-five, or drink more than two alcoholic beverages daily. The longer you stay on the pill, the greater your odds of becoming hypertensive.

Why does this happen? Estrogen triggers the production of aldosterone, a hormone that promotes sodium retention and increased plasma volume. The increased plasma volume is responsible for the weight gain or bloating experienced by most women who take the pill. In addition, as the plasma volume expands, a woman's cardiac output increases. In other words, her heart has to work harder to pump the extra fluid, which in turn raises her blood pressure. During pregnancy, the cardiovascular system cooperates by dilating or opening up to accommodate the increased plasma volume. But when a woman is on the pill, this intricate network of arteries and blood vessels actually works against her. The muscle tone of the small arteries increases, and the cells on the vessel walls thicken, which makes them stiffer and more resistant to the flow of blood. (Oddly enough, although women who take ERT postmenopausally may have an increased aldosterone secretion, it does not raise their blood pressure.)

Oral contraceptives also appear to make a woman more prone to develop cardiovascular disease. Although the rate of death from coronary disease is declining, users of oral contraceptives risk a threefold increase in death from cardiovascular disease and a sevenfold increase in cerebral vascular death or stroke. Studies show that women who smoke and take the pill run a 40 percent greater risk of developing cardiovascular disease. To put this statistic in context, consider the fact that under the best of circumstances one out of two women will eventually die of CAD. Increasing that risk by 40 percent makes death by CAD even more likely.

Another negative side effect of the pill includes an increased tendency on the part of some women to form blood clots. In addition, some women on the pill complain of increased irritability and depression—not unlike the mood swings experienced by some women during their monthly menstrual cycle. Women prone to migraines may suffer an increased incidence of these troublesome headaches on the pill.

There are also some significant adverse changes in fat and carbohydrate metabolism reported in some pill users. Estrogen raises triglyceride levels, which in women, puts them at greater risk of developing CAD. Progestin raises LDL levels and decreases the beneficial HDL, thus increasing the woman's risk of developing arteriosclerosis. From a cardiovascular point of view, however, some progestins are more dangerous than others. One study showed that progestins that are both highly potent and androgenic, that is, more likely to promote male characteristics, have a much worse effect on lipids than progestins that are not androgenic. The study compared two commonly used low-dose estrogen pills, Ovcon 35, which does not contain the highly androgenic progestins, and Lo/Ovral, which does. According to the researchers, users of Ovcon 35 had a mild increase in LDLs, and a beneficial increase in HDLs, while users of Lo/Ovral had elevated LDLs and lowered HDLs. The study shows that not all birth control pills are the same. If you do take the pill, it's important to talk to your gynecologist about selecting the right one for you.

In all fairness to the pill, many of these negative findings were based on studies of women who were using higher doses of estrogen than are commonly in vogue: 50 micrograms of the hormone versus the 20 to 35 micrograms used in many pills today. We simply don't know yet, however, if the lower estrogen dose will prove to be any safer in the long run.

After reading all of these negative findings, some women on oral contraceptives may feel like dropping their package of pills down the nearest incinerator. Don't do it. Although I am the first to say that the pill is not for everyone, there are many women who can take it safely and with a minimum of side effects. In addition, there are many women who manage to take the pill every day who would not be as conscientious about using other forms of birth control. Keep in mind that there are also risks involved in pregnancy, especially in unplanned pregnancies terminated by abortion.

Women who should not even consider taking the pill are those who are already hypertensive or who developed hypertension in a previous pregnancy, women who are overweight, or women who smoke. I cannot stress enough that women who smoke do not belong on the pill.

Prior to taking the pill, I recommend that every woman have a complete physical exam that includes the following:

1. A lipid profile including total cholesterol screening, as well as a breakdown of HDL, LDL, and triglycerides. If a woman's three-times-tested fasting levels of cholesterol are over 220 mg/dl, or if her triglycerides are over 190 mg/dl, I do not believe she should be given the pill.
2. A blood pressure check. Women with elevated blood pressures should not be on the pill.
3. A review of the risks of birth control pills. All patients must be warned against smoking.

If your doctor decides that you are a good candidate for the pill, your first prescription should be for no more than three months. After that, you should return to your doctor for a complete examination before your prescription is renewed. At that time, your doctor should recheck your blood pressure. He should also look for any weight gain or swelling of your feet to rule out excessive water retention. If you find that you have to use diuretics or water pills to reduce edema, quit using the pill. Your doctor should ask if you've had any headaches, unusual mood changes, or palpitations. (If he doesn't ask, and you've had any of these symptoms, be sure to tell him.) If you've experienced any of these unpleasant and potentially dangerous side effects, you and your doctor should discuss alternative forms of contraception. If you're a pill user, be sure to visit your doctor every six months, at which point he should do a complete physical examination and repeat the blood lipid profile.

Chapter 4

PREGNANCY
AND YOUR HEART

IF you think that pregnancy only involves your reproductive organs, you're wrong. Your heart—in fact, your entire cardiovascular system—is a major player throughout the pregnancy and childbirth process.

From a cardiovascular point of view, pregnancy and childbirth are a lot like climbing Mt. Everest. During the nine months of pregnancy, culminating in labor and delivery, your heart will have to work harder than it has ever worked before, or probably will ever have to work again. Your heart must respond to the dramatic changes that are occurring throughout your body, from the moment of conception, right up until the first time you cuddle your newborn in your arms.

During pregnancy, your body produces increased amounts of two critical hormones: progesterone and estrogen. Without these chemicals you would not be able to make the necessary adjustments to support the new life growing inside your uterus. The increased levels of these hormones are responsible for many of the physical and emotional changes women often experience during pregnancy. Nausea or the infamous "morning sickness," prevalent during the first trimester, is due to sudden changes in hormonal levels. Swelling of the breasts, constipation, insomnia, and increased urination, so common later in pregnancy, are also orchestrated largely by these potent chemicals.

Perhaps the greatest changes of all are the ones that are occurring in your cardiovascular system. Some of them you may actually feel, but some you may not.

To meet the demands of pregnancy, the mother-to-be's blood volume—the fluid portion of her blood—eventually increases by nearly 50 percent. The increased blood volume is necessary to provide adequate support to the fetus, who relies solely on the mother for nourishment. The developing baby gets vital nutrients and oxygen through the umbilical cord. The cord is attached to the placenta, a remarkable organ that is created solely to support the pregnancy. Since it is expelled immediately after birth, it is sometimes called the "afterbirth." Oxygen and nutrients flow in one direction, while carbon dioxide and fetal waste flow in another. The extra blood volume serves two purposes: It supplies the placenta with oxygen and nutrients, and also ensures that the mother's body is not being deprived of those same things in the process.

The expanded blood volume does another important job: It helps keep temperature constant throughout the body. During pregnancy, a woman's body shifts into overdrive. To accomplish the growing workload, the mother's metabolism—the rate at which she converts food to energy and other substances needed to maintain life—speeds up. To provide the fuel needed to perform the work, her body requires increased amounts of the basic elements of life: food, water, and oxygen.

Every organ, from the heart to the kidneys, works about 50 percent harder to meet the needs of both the mother and the baby. The harder everything works, the more heat is generated. This is true not only of the mother's body but also of the baby's. As the fetus grows and becomes more active, it must also lose heat through the mother's circulation. The mother's expanded blood volume helps cool down the body. Even with this added help, many pregnant women often complain of being too warm, even during the coldest days of winter.

How does the heart adapt to the demands of pregnancy? The heart's job is to pump enough blood throughout the body to feed all the organs and tissues, from the head to the toes. Until about the twentieth week, the heart compensates for pregnancy by pumping more blood with each beat or stroke. By the third trimester, however, when the blood volume has reached its peak, the heart beats faster to circulate the extra liquid.

When the heart pumps a greater volume of fluid, more blood pulses through the body's vast network of arteries, veins, and capillaries. Under normal circumstances, this extra fluid would cause a myriad of problems. The heart could be overwhelmed. The blood that the heart could not pump forward would back up and fluid would accumulate in the lungs. This is called heart failure; eventually the organ can simply stop beating. But that doesn't happen.

Fortunately, the mother-to-be has adapted to this situation, thanks to the production of two chemicals called prostaglandins. These substances work in unison to accommodate the increased blood flow, but in opposite ways. The first, prostacyclin, relaxes the blood vessels, causing them to expand or dilate, thus accommodating the increased blood volume of pregnancy. In the process, it lowers the blood pressure. But prostacyclin by itself would leave the blood vessels too relaxed. That's where the second prostaglandin, thromboxane A_2, enters the picture. Thromboxane A_2 actually raises the blood pressure by causing the smooth muscle cells in the walls of the blood vessels to constrict or narrow.

A delicate balance of both prostaglandins is needed to maintain normal blood pressure during pregnancy. Too much of either can cause serious problems. Thromboxane A_2 also has another critical role. It activates the blood platelets by making them more prone to coagulation or clotting, probably to prevent maternal hemorrhaging during delivery when the placenta separates from the baby.

Toward the end of pregnancy, as the baby grows and the uterus enlarges, it becomes increasingly difficult for mothers-to-be to get around. Many women find that they are frequently short of breath after even the slightest exertion. The growing uterus is pressing down on the diaphragm, making it difficult for the mother to fully expand her lungs to get enough oxygen. At the same time, hormonal changes have made the circulatory system more sensitive to hypoxia, or oxygen deprivation, probably to ensure that the fetus gets enough of this vital element. As soon as the mother's level of oxygen dips even slightly, she will begin to hyperventilate, or take in short, rapid breaths. As a result, even women who used practically to leap up a flight of stairs in a single bound may now find themselves huffing and puffing after a few steps.

Many pregnant women also notice that some resting positions are better than others. For instance, when they lie on their backs, they may feel uncomfortable and even light-headed. In this position, the growing uterus falls directly on the inferior vena cava, the great vessel that drains the whole lower body, returning the blood from the lower body to the right side of the heart. If the work of the vena cava is hampered, fluid may collect in the lower extremities, causing the edema or swelling that is so common in pregnancy. Support hose can help keep the blood flowing. Frequently elevating your feet throughout the day can also help. Lying on your side relieves pressure on the vena cava and will actually increase the blood flow to the placenta. This position is beneficial to both mother and baby.

By the third trimester, the mother's electrocardiogram will show some variation of the norm due to the fact that the heart itself shifts its position. The enlarged abdomen is pressing against the diaphragm, which in turn lifts the heart into a more horizontal position in the chest. If you listen to the heart with a stethoscope, you will hear an extra sound called a murmur that is caused by the unusually large volume of blood flowing through the heart with each beat.

One of the most exciting moments of pregnancy occurs around the sixth week of gestation when the expectant mother may be able to hear the beating of her baby's heart. A Doppler, a hand-held ultrasound device, can detect a heartbeat at around six weeks after conception for some, but not all, babies.

Since babies develop at different rates inside the womb, it may take longer to find a heartbeat for some babies than for others.

Because her heart is working so much harder, a woman may be more aware of her heart during pregnancy than at any other time in her life. She is very likely to experience very rapid beats or palpitations and even occasional arrhythmias. And it is not unusual for a mother-to-be sometimes to feel as if her heart is racing in her chest. After all, her heart is working overtime maintaining two (or in the case of multiple births, even more) lives. For many women, pregnancy also exacts an emotional toll. Anxiety—not uncommon during pregnancy—can actually increase cardiac output and place an added strain on an already overburdened heart.

Some women may be concerned about the impending delivery; others are worried about juggling the demands of a career and a family. If you are feeling overwhelmed, or are under a lot of stress during pregnancy, it's important to talk about your fears with your doctor or, if necessary, a therapist. Short-term therapy can often yield long-term benefits. A case in point is one recent study of pregnant women who developed a rapid heartbeat due to anxiety. After receiving appropriate counseling, these women reduced their heart rate by 20 percent without having to take any medication! To me, that underscores the importance of having a doctor with whom you feel comfortable and can talk honestly.

Most women will be able to meet the challenge of pregnancy with few if any problems. However, there are some serious cardiac conditions that can complicate a pregnancy. Sometimes they strike without warning, but more often than not, they are missed or ignored. Sometimes even seemingly benign symptoms can actually be a sign of a greater problem. Too often, however, any discomfort or unusual symptoms experienced by a pregnant woman are cavalierly dismissed by both the woman and her physician as normal aches and pains of pregnancy. Therefore, it is essential that all women are made aware of these possible problems, and even more importantly, that their physicians treat their complaints seriously.

PREGNANCY AND HEART DISEASE

Most women can easily tolerate the added burden of pregnancy. But for women with preexisting or undiagnosed heart conditions, it's a different story. In some cases, pregnancy can pose a serious risk—and in rare cases, it shouldn't even be considered. With proper medical attention, however, many women with heart problems, including damaged valves and congenital heart defects, can safely have children.

If you have a heart problem, talk to your doctor before getting pregnant. She will be able to assess your chances of having a successful pregnancy. Once pregnant, you will probably require closer monitoring than other patients. In addition, you should be treated by someone who is experienced in cases such as your own.

Any woman who has had rheumatic heart disease should be especially careful during pregnancy. Rheumatic heart disease begins innocently enough with strep throat (an infection of the throat due to a bacteria called streptococcus) or with scarlet fever, which is caused by the same bacteria. Symptoms of strep include:

1. Swollen glands
2. Difficulty swallowing
3. Fever

If a streptococcal infection goes untreated, it may be followed by acute rheumatic fever, which can eventually damage and scar the heart valves. Although people of any age can get rheumatic fever, it usually strikes between the ages of five and fifteen. Some victims of rheumatic fever will get very sick, suffering from telltale signs such as high fever, chest pains, and shortness of breath, indicating that the heart has been affected. Unfortunately, some cases go undiagnosed because the only symptom may have been a mild sore throat. However, during a subsequent physical examination, a good doctor should be able to detect any unusual murmurs or heart sounds that may indicate any scarrings or malfunctions of the heart and valves. Diagnosis prior to pregnancy is critical for the health and well-being of the mother and child. When a woman with rheumatic heart disease is confronted with the added physical strain of pregnancy, she is at risk of developing cardiac complications, if she has not done so already.

One of the most serious lesions of rheumatic heart disease is mitral stenosis, a condition in which the mitral valve, which guards the exit from the left atrium into the left ventricle, is scarred, thickened, and distorted by the body's response to the streptococcal infection. If there is a severe enough narrowing of the scarred valve, blood may back up in the lungs, which can cause pulmonary edema or the flooding of the air spaces of the lungs with fluid. In some cases, it can lead to sudden death. Signs of mitral stenosis include:

1. Coughing due to fluid buildup in the lungs. (Earlier in the course of the congestion, the fluid is clear, but may later become pink with blood.)
2. Shortness of breath.
3. Fatigue.

The last two symptoms can easily be masked by the normal symptoms of pregnancy.

In other cases, the aortic valve—the one guarding the opening of the left ventricle into the aorta—is the one that has been injured. The valve leaflets may have become partially fused and stiff, constricting the exit from the chamber, resulting in a condition called aortic stenosis. In other cases, the leaflets may have become so distorted that they allow the blood to flow backward from the aorta into the left ventricle. Since the first arteries branching from the aorta are the coronary arteries, scarring of the aortic valve may deprive the heart of good blood flow through those arteries. The heart may suffer oxygen deprivation, leading to symptoms of angina or chest pain, and in severe cases, congestive heart failure. Symptoms of aortic stenosis include:

1. Shortness of breath, panting, or difficulty breathing
2. Fainting

Once again, all these symptoms could be dismissed as "normal" side effects of pregnancy by both the woman and her physician.

In cases of aortic stenosis, the defective valve must be replaced, preferably before pregnancy. If the surgery is performed during pregnancy, there is a 30 percent chance of fetal death, probably due to oxygen deprivation. Women who have artificial valves run a higher risk of clotting during pregnancy and usually require an anticoagulant drug such as heparin, which does not cross the placenta. Women of childbearing age should be given valves derived from animal tissue, which reduce their risk of clotting and may even eliminate the need for other medication.

Women who have had rheumatic heart disease must be given antibiotics during labor and shortly after delivery to guard against bacterial endocarditis, an infection that can attack the damaged and vulnerable leaflets of affected valves.

In the case of rheumatic heart disease, of course your best bet is to avoid getting it in the first place. If you have a sore throat, have it cultured by your doctor to detect the strep infection. If it is positive for strep, take a prescribed antibiotic. And if you or your child have a fever for more than two days, call your doctor. If your doctor suspects rheumatic fever, he may order an EKG or other diagnostic studies to detect whether or not the heart has been adversely affected.

If you suspect that you've had rheumatic heart disease, before you get pregnant you should have a thorough physical examination by a competent physician who will check for any abnormalities of the valves or of the heart muscle itself.

ANEMIA

Anemia is one of the most common ailments of pregnancy. Although it is rarely life-threatening, it can be extremely debilitating. I know from firsthand experience. When I was pregnant with my daughter, my obstetrician advised me simply to eat a well-balanced diet and let nature take care of the rest. We never actually discussed what a well-balanced diet was, or how a woman's nutritional needs change during pregnancy. He didn't even prescribe a vitamin supplement. I continued to eat exactly the same way as I had before my pregnancy: a bowl of cereal and a cup of coffee for breakfast, a quick sandwich and a glass of milk for lunch, and whatever I had the strength to throw together for dinner when I got home from the hospital.

By the fifth month of pregnancy, I felt so exhausted that I was unable to summon up the strength to get out of bed in the morning. I remember thinking that each step I took was like trying to walk under water—it took tremendous effort simply to move one foot in front of the other. Not only that, but I looked terrible. My normally rosy complexion was pale and gray. I knew that many women often complained of feeling tired during pregnancy, but I also knew that the sheer exhaustion that I was experiencing could not be normal. I called my doctor and described my symptoms. He wanted to see me immediately. As I had suspected, something was wrong. A blood smear examined under a microscope revealed that I was producing fewer, larger, and more immature red blood cells—a classic sign of folate deficiency anemia. In addition, a blood test revealed that my hemoglobin or red blood cell count had dipped to 6 grams, whereas a normal level would have been around 12 grams.

When I learned my diagnosis, I realized why I had been feeling so run-down. Folic acid is a B vitamin that plays an essential role in the production of red blood cells. It is also necessary for the production of DNA, the so-called building blocks of the body. A pregnant woman needs about 800 milligrams of folic acid daily—double the normal amount—in order to produce enough blood cells to meet the needs of herself and her baby. Red blood cells are important because they contain hemoglobin, which carries oxygen throughout the mother's body and to the baby via the placenta. If the mother does not produce enough red blood cells to do the job, her heart will have to pump more blood to supply enough oxygen to her body and the placenta. And she will feel very, very draggy and tired.

Women who suffer from a folate deficiency during pregnancy are usually advised to take a folate supplement. They must also eat more foods rich in this precious element. Organ meats, eggs, and leafy green vegetables top the list. A daily vitamin supplement and better nutrition did the trick for me. Within just a week, I felt like a new woman.

There are several reasons why women are more prone to anemia during pregnancy than at other times in their lives. As we have said, during pregnancy the mother's blood volume increases by a whopping 50 percent, yet her production of red cells increases by only 30 percent. The low red blood cell to blood volume ratio is sometimes called the "physiologic" anemia of pregnancy. It is perfectly normal for an expectant mother's hematocrit, or the total percent of red blood cells in the blood, to be slightly lower than usual. However, it is critical that her doctor closely monitor her blood count so it doesn't fall so low that she becomes truly anemic. Based on my own experience, I advise women to have their blood count checked monthly by their physicians, and even more frequently if they begin to experience extreme tiredness or fatigue. Needless to say, I am also a strong advocate of taking a vitamin supplement during pregnancy as long as it is prescribed by your doctor. It is especially critical for women who have been using oral contraceptives prior to pregnancy, since estrogen can deplete folate reserves. These women should talk to their doctors about taking additional supplements beyond those that are usually prescribed.

Iron deficiency anemia is another common malady of pregnancy. And no wonder. Iron is also essential in the production of the hemoglobin contained in red blood cells. Iron deficiency may not only result in extreme fatigue but may cause a decreased tolerance for blood loss during delivery and a greater susceptibility for infection. Since the baby also needs iron for the production of red blood cells, she will "rob" from maternal stores if she's not getting enough from the mother's blood supply. Toward the end of the third trimester, the baby will sap even more iron from the mother as she builds up her own supply. She will need this extra iron during the first few months of life, when her main source of nourishment is milk, a poor source of this essential element.

Most pregnant women are given iron supplements by their doctors. It is especially critical for women to take supplements if they entered pregnancy with low iron reserves. Women who have had heavy menstrual periods, or who have a history of anemia, should ask their doctors about additional supplements. Do not take any iron supplement without first consulting your doctor, since an overdose can have a toxic effect on the fetus.

It is, however, perfectly safe to increase your iron intake by eating foods rich in this vital element. Liver, red meat, dark green vegetables, and whole grains can help maintain adequate iron reserves. Iron in food is better absorbed if taken along with a vitamin C source at the same meal, such as orange juice or broccoli. Since iron supplements can sometimes cause stomach irritation, it's better to take them during meals than on an empty stomach.

You may be surprised that a physician recommends cholesterol-rich food such as liver or red meat. But during pregnancy, the extra cholesterol is put to good use. Cholesterol is essential in the production of new cells. Your developing baby needs cholesterol to grow properly. In fact, during pregnancy your cholesterol level could rise by as much as 30 percent, but it will return to normal by the twentieth week postpartum. If you're beginning your pregnancy with a cholesterol level within normal limits, feel free to indulge in a slice of liver or a piece of steak every night without fretting over your LDL/HDL ratio. However, if you're starting a pregnancy with a total cholesterol level of 240 or higher, talk to your doctor about dietary guidelines. Depending on other risk factors, he may advise a modified diet that is low in cholesterol.

Pregnancy is an amazing process. It begins with one single cell. About 266 days—or 200 million cells later—a baby is ready to be born. In order for the process to work, for the baby to grow properly and for the mother to maintain her health, a pregnant women must be adequately nourished. A well-balanced diet designed to meet the increased nutritional needs of pregnancy, and a vitamin supplement, can make a real difference in the way a pregnant woman looks and feels.

PREECLAMPSIA, OR PREGNANCY-INDUCED HYPERTENSION

When I was an intern working in the emergency room of one of New York's busiest hospitals, I would frequently see women with pregnancy-induced hypertension, or preeclampsia. These cases were especially compelling because two lives were at stake: the mother's and the baby's.

Blood pressure levels usually drop by the middle of pregnancy to below 120/80 and bounce back to normal before delivery. The 120 measures the pressure in the arteries when the heart is contracting: It is the systolic pressure. The 80 represents the pressure in the arteries when the heart is relaxed: It is the diastolic pressure. However, about 7 percent of all mothers-to-be develop preeclampsia, or pregnancy-induced hypertension, characterized by high blood pressure, excessive swelling, and protein in the urine. Since most women experience some swelling during pregnancy, a danger sign may be shoes or gloves that suddenly no longer fit.

Preeclampsia can be dangerous to both mother and child. If untreated, it can develop into a full-blown case of maternal eclampsia, an extremely serious condition that can lead to convulsions, failure of various organ systems, coma, and even maternal death. An already overworked heart trying to cope with the normal volume overload of pregnancy now has to work even harder to pump enough blood and oxygen throughout the body. Since the mother's blood vessels are constricted in the hypertensive state, the blood flow to the uterus becomes impaired. It can result in a malnourished and oxygen-deprived fetus.

If the fetus is not properly nourished, she cannot develop and grow properly. In some cases, the baby may have to be delivered before term, putting her at risk of a whole host of other problems resulting from a premature departure from the womb. In extreme cases, the blood vessels leading to the placenta may weaken, causing the placenta to tear away from the uterine wall, causing a condition called abruptio placentae. Abruptio placentae can lead to maternal bleeding, hemorrhaging, and premature birth.

Preeclampsia typically strikes during a first pregnancy, although it can happen in later ones. The problem typically does not appear until the second trimester—usually around the twentieth week—when the maternal blood volume is reaching its peak. Women who are at greatest risk include expectant mothers over thirty-five, diabetics or those with a family history of this disorder, or women who are overweight. High-risk women should be especially vigilant about monitoring their blood pressure during pregnancy. In fact, their doctors may recommend that they purchase an inexpensive blood-pressure gauge to monitor their pressure at home. It's also important to remember that preeclampsia can happen to any pregnant woman and for this reason it is a good idea for all women to know the symptoms.

Although preeclampsia sometimes develops without any warning, often there are subtle signs that indicate a problem is brewing:

1. Sudden weight gain of more than 2 pounds in any given week, accompanied by unusual swelling of hands, feet, or lower legs
2. A headache that doesn't go away within a few hours
3. Pain in the upper abdomen
4. Blurred vision or dizziness

If you experience any of these symptoms, call your doctor immediately.

Now that I've told you the bad news, the good news is that if it is caught early, mild preeclampsia can usually be controlled and the mother can carry her baby safely to term. Very often, the only treatment that may be necessary is increased rest and improved nutrition. A woman with this problem is usually advised to lie on her left side several times a day to help improve circulation to her uterus and other vital organs. She should avoid lying on her back, because in the supine position, as we have explained, the growing uterus will compress the inferior cava. If "natural" solutions don't bring down the blood pressure, antihypertensive medication may be required. (No medication should be taken during pregnancy unless it is under a doctor's supervision.)

The cause of pregnancy-induced hypertension is still a mystery, although researchers have come up with some promising theories. As we discussed earlier, two hormones are produced during pregnancy that have a direct effect on the blood vessels: thromboxane A_2 and prostacyclin. Thromboxane causes the vessels to constrict while prostacyclin counteracts the thromboxane by causing the vessels to expand or dilate. Some researchers believe that hypertension occurs when there is an improper imbalance of thromboxane and prostacyclin, so that the vessels remain too constricted.

Is it possible to prevent pregnancy-induced hypertension from developing in the first place? Since we don't know for sure what causes the problem, we can't be certain how to prevent it. Obviously, eliminating major risk factors such as obesity, eating a well-balanced diet during pregnancy, and keeping appointments with your obstetrician may help reduce your chances of developing hypertension.

Some women, however, especially those who are obese or already hypertensive, may need to take special measures to prevent the onset of preeclampsia. Two recent studies in the *New England Journal of Medicine* recommended the use of low daily doses of aspirin as a means to reduce significantly the incidence of hypertension during pregnancy. Aspirin, an antiprostaglandin, probably inhibits the production of thromboxane, which in turn prevents the vessels from constricting. According to the studies, high-risk women treated with aspirin in the third trimester carried longer and delivered higher birth-weight babies than high-risk women who did not take aspirin.

However, there are some potentially dangerous side effects. Thromboxane also activates the platelets for clotting in preparation for delivery. If aspirin interferes with the production of thromboxane, it could increase the risk of maternal bleeding. There is also an increased risk of fetal hemorrhaging if the aspirin is taken up to five days prior to delivery. Other animal studies suggest that exposure to antiprostaglandins such as aspirin *in utero* could induce major cardiovascular changes in the fetus, including the premature closure of one particular blood vessel, the ductus arteriosus. Such closure could cause fetal heart failure.

Despite the potential negative side effects, the use of aspirin to prevent hypertension during pregnancy is an exciting development. If you are a woman who is at high risk of developing pregnancy-induced hypertension, perhaps you should discuss the possible use of aspirin with your obstetrician.

When it comes to preeclampsia, prevention is the best medicine. Good prenatal nutrition, adequate rest, and proper medical care can help prevent this potentially life-threatening disorder.

PERIPARTUM CARDIOMYOPATHY

A cardiomyopathy (literally, "heart muscle illness") is a primary lesion of the heart muscle. In women who develop this problem, parts of the heart are damaged. The healthy areas of the ventricle will still continue to pump normally, but those that are not healthy will balloon outward or not contract at all when the rest of the chamber works normally. The ventricle cannot pump blood efficiently, and congestive heart failure may result. Symptoms of peripartum cardiomyopathy include:

1. Exhaustion at the slightest exertion
2. Shortness of breath
3. Tachycardia, or fast heartbeat
4. Inability to sleep lying flat on your back
5. Swelling of the feet

What causes the peripartum cardiomyopathy? Interestingly enough, proteins produced by the mother's own body may be the culprit. During the last month of pregnancy, the uterus, in preparation for labor and delivery, releases certain contractile proteins into the bloodstream from its muscle cells. These proteins are not normally found in the blood but are confined by cell membranes in all types of muscle cells throughout the body. In fact, uterine muscle proteins are chemically similar to two virtually identical contractile proteins in the heart cells: actin and myosin.

Most women are able to tolerate small amounts of uterine proteins in their bloodstream. However, some women cannot—they do not recognize these proteins as being part of themselves; rather they view them as intruders. Once it spots the uterine proteins, their body begins to produce other proteins called antibodies to attack the "invading" proteins. Since the uterine proteins are so similar to proteins found in the heart, the body also directs the antibodies against heart cells. As a result of their attack, the heart muscle softens and dilates. If the damage is severe enough, the heart fails. The process is called an autoimmune reaction: The body does not recognize parts of its own tissues.

Peripartum cardiomyopathy can be treated with rest, improved diet, salt restriction, and in some cases, immunosuppressive drugs, which are drugs that suppress the production of antibodies.

Depending on whose figures you believe, this condition occurs in anywhere from 1 out of 4,000 to 1 out of 15,000 pregnancies. Women who are over thirty-five, carrying twins, malnourished, or hypertensive are at greatest risk of developing a cardiomyopathy. Surprisingly, once pregnancy is over, the process stops. If the damage has not been too great, the size and function of the left ventricle returns to normal within six months after delivery. In such cases, the prognosis is good for future pregnancies, but there is also a strong chance for recurrence. Therefore, I think that any woman who has experienced this problem should think very carefully before embarking on a future pregnancy. If she decides to go ahead with it anyway, she should be especially vigilant about monitoring her blood pressure during pregnancy, eating well, and getting enough rest. Most importantly, she should work closely with a qualified obstetrician who is familiar with her problem.

SMOKING

As a physician who has treated smokers for more than thirty years, I know that it is very tough to quit. Through the years, I have learned two important lessons: You can't reform a smoker who doesn't want to be reformed, and only the most motivated people will actually kick the habit.

For many women, pregnancy provides the motivation needed to endure the discomfort of quitting. About one-third of all women who become pregnant are smokers. To their credit, about one-quarter of these women stop smoking at some point during their pregnancy. Three-quarters of all women smokers, however, continue to puff away the entire time their baby is growing inside their womb.

Pregnancy may be a mere nine months of a woman's life, but it is a critical period for her unborn child. A new human being is being created inside the uterus. This potential life relies on the mother for everything needed to grow properly, including oxygen and vital nutrients. A woman who smokes is shortchanging her child of these precious life supports. The evidence against smoking during pregnancy is overwhelming. Smokers have increased levels of carbon monoxide in their blood, thus making less oxygen available to their tissues. They also have higher blood levels of carbon dioxide, which passes through the placenta, thus robbing the flow of oxygen to the fetal tissues— oxygen needed not only for maintenance but for proper growth.

The nicotine in tobacco causes blood vessels to constrict—including those of the placenta—which interferes with the flow of nutrients through the placenta to the fetus. As a result, the babies of smokers weigh on average 7 ounces less than the babies of nonsmokers. In fact, about one-third of all cases of low birth-weight babies—under 5.5 pounds—are born to smoker-mothers. Underweight infants run a greater risk of stillbirth and neonatal death. Also, the babies of women smokers are at increased risk of dying from crib death or sudden infant death syndrome (SIDS).

Women who smoke are more likely to develop complications such as spontaneous abortion, abruptio placentae (a premature separation of the placenta from the uterine wall) or placenta previa (a condition in which the placenta is poorly situated inside the uterine cavity, growing over all or part of the cervix, the opening of the womb into the vagina.)

Smoking hurts the baby inside the womb in other ways. Although unborn babies don't really breathe, they do practice some motions of breathing by exercising certain chest muscles. Studies show that after just two cigarettes, a baby's chest movements slow down.

A mother's smoking may not just affect life in the womb but may have long-term consequences. According to some studies, children of mothers who smoked during pregnancy score lower on math and verbal tests than those of nonsmokers.

All in all, maternal smoking during pregnancy may lead to 5,000 extra and entirely avoidable perinatal deaths per year, that is, fetal deaths that occur in the eight weeks prior to birth or infant death up to seven days after birth.

Even after the baby is born, she is not immune to the hazards of maternal smoking. Breathing smoke in the nursery can be every bit as damaging as exposure in the womb. During the first year of life, children whose parents smoke have a higher rate of pneumonia and bronchitis than children of nonsmokers. And if either you or your spouse smokes, don't be surprised to find a pack of cigarettes on your child when he or she reaches adolescence. As a mother of two, I can tell you that children do as you do, not as you say.

Quitting is difficult but not impossible. A few brave souls can go cold turkey, but many people need extra help. I often suggest that patients contact Smokenders or the smoking cessation program run by the American Lung Association.

Also, talk to your obstetrician about establishing a support group for pregnant women who are trying to quit smoking. Together, you can give each other the strength to overcome a dangerous and life-threatening addiction.

III

WHAT CAN GO WRONG

Chapter 5

CORONARY
ARTERY DISEASE

MY patient Betsy, a fifty-four-year-old interior designer, noticed that she could no longer play tennis without getting so winded that she'd have to sit down to catch her breath after just a few volleys. When she told me about her problem, I recommended that she have a few diagnostic tests to see if her symptoms could be related to her heart. The test results confirmed my suspicions: Betsy had coronary artery disease (CAD), a narrowing in one of the coronary arteries that provides blood and oxygen to the heart. Fortunately, I was able to treat Betsy with Procardia, one of several types of drugs that help to dilate the coronary arteries, allowing the blood to flow more freely. Both her tennis game and her life have vastly improved. Nevertheless, I watch Betsy very carefully—as I do all my patients with CAD—because this disease is the number one killer of women (and men) in the United States.

When we talk about the lethal effects of CAD, we're really talking about the devastating effect of the process called arteriosclerosis, that occurs when arteries become clogged with a thick, yellowish, waxy substance called plaque, impeding the flow of blood to body organs. Plaque consists of a variety of cells including cholesterol, a fat or lipid that is primarily produced in the liver.

Arteriosclerosis is a progressive disease that may begin as early as infancy, although it may take decades for symptoms to appear. Usually, these are angina, or chest pain, and/or shortness of breath upon mild exertion. There is no cure for arteriosclerosis. Although we can treat it in a variety of ways, including medication, and in severe cases, surgery, we have not been able to take a diseased artery and restore it completely to its original state. If the arteries feeding the heart become so clogged with plaque that they cannot deliver enough oxygen and vital nutrients to the heart, portions of the muscle will die or suffer irreparable damage. Severe damage can be life-threatening. If arteries supplying blood to the brain become blocked, the resulting damage can cause a stroke, or death of brain tissue.

About half of all women in the United States will die of diseases directly related to arteriosclerosis. Many researchers—myself included—believe that a diet high in cholesterol and saturated fat and high blood cholesterol levels play a role in the development of this disease. In recent years, however, there has been a great deal of controversy over the relationship between cholesterol and arteriosclerosis. On the one hand, the American Heart Association and the federally funded National Heart, Lung and Blood Institute are cosponsoring the National Cholesterol Education Program, a campaign to reduce blood cholesterol levels across the country. On the other hand, a few physicians question whether the program is overemphasizing the importance of total cholesterol as a risk factor while ignoring others.

Other critics question the entire diet–cholesterol–heart disease link, claiming that it has not been conclusively proven in humans that a high-fat diet raises the risk of CAD. Still others debate whether any of this discussion applies to women at all, since women have been excluded from the major intervention studies designed to test the cholesterol theory. Therefore, some go as far as to suggest that women don't need to have their cholesterol tested, nor do they need to follow the dietary guidelines designed to lower cholesterol.

These critics have a point. Doctors should not blindly follow male treatment models for women patients. There are biological differences between men and women that should be considered when treating CAD. For one thing, a blood cholesterol level that is dangerous for men may not be so for women. Similarly, there are other blood lipids that, if too high, are particularly lethal for women but do not seem to be so for men. I strongly disagree, however, with critics who say that women need not worry about diet or cholesterol at all. An examination of the facts makes a compelling case against a high-fat diet for both sexes. And although cholesterol is not the only risk factor for CAD, it is still an important one.

Women need to know what the cholesterol debate is all about, and more importantly, how it affects their lives. Once you understand the disease process, you will be able to review the facts critically and come to your own conclusion. You will understand why arteriosclerosis is so difficult to control and why, despite all of our best efforts, it is still the leading cause of death in the United States. You will also understand why so many physicians believe that prevention may be our best weapon against this disease.

In chapter 1, we saw that the heart is a hardworking muscle composed of about two billion tiny individual units called myocytes or cells. Myocytes are cells that work in unison to keep the heart pumping and the blood flowing throughout the body. Like all tissues, the working heart itself needs blood to carry out its work. When the coronary arteries are diseased—as they are in arteriosclerosis—blood flow to this important muscle can become inadequate to nourish the heart. To understand fully what arteriosclerosis is, and the conditions that breed this potentially deadly disease, you must first have some idea of the actual structure of an artery.

If you sliced open an artery, as you would slice a sausage, and put the slice under a microscope, you would see layers of concentric circles, similar to those of an onion. At the core of the artery is the lumen, the passageway through which the blood flows. The lumen is surrounded by a single layer of cells called the endothelium, a major player in the development of arteriosclerosis. The endothelium is surrounded by the intima. Outside the intimal layer is an important layer called the media, primarily composed of specialized muscle cells. They, too, are essential players in what often turns out to be a struggle for life or death. The two outer layers—the external elastic lamella, and covering it, the tunica adventitia—complete the arterial wall. It's not important to memorize the names of all the layers, but it is important that you understand that an artery contains several layers of different types of cells that belong in specific places. Problems can arise when some of these cells migrate out of their proper neighborhoods to places where they don't belong.

Arteriosclerosis probably begins in the endothelium, the single layer of cells surrounding the lumen, the inner core of the artery through which the blood flows. The endothelium is a very thin protective barrier about 1/1,000 of the width of a human hair. Just as the thinnest layer of polish protects furniture

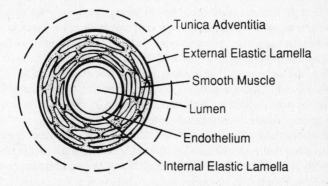

Tunica Adventitia

External Elastic Lamella

Smooth Muscle

Lumen

Endothelium

Internal Elastic Lamella

INSIDE VIEW OF AN ARTERY

against moisture and dust, the endothelial cells protect the artery from un-wanted guests that may float in the blood. Because they are so thin, the endothelial cells can be easily damaged, and in most cases, they can quickly repair themselves. If the injury is too severe and the cells cannot heal in time, neighboring cells from other parts of the artery fill the void. Smooth muscle cells from the media migrate to the intima, the layer surrounding the endothelium—and that's where the trouble begins.

When smooth cells move to the intima, they begin to multiply rapidly and also to attract other cells, including lipids or fats. This situation is the begin-ning of the formation of plaque, a lesion that has many components including cholesterol, smooth muscle cells, and special scavenger cells called foam cells. Over time, the expanding plaque lesion grows large enough to obstruct the flow of blood either partially or completely. In advanced lesions, pieces of the plaque or the blood clots that stick to it can break off and block vessels further downstream. In the case of larger arteries, such as the aorta, advanced arteriosclerosis can even destroy portions of the artery wall, resulting in a weakened, stretched spot called an aneurysm. If the process continues, it can produce an actual rupture of the wall.

There are two excellent theories of why arteriosclerosis develops, but we still have no definitive answers. The first, known as the injury response theory, proposes that the arteriosclerotic process is actually a result of an injury to the endothelium, the protective layer around the arterial lumen. Injury is defined very liberally to mean anything that can disturb the normal function of the cell. For instance, an injury could be any change in the permeability of the cell, which means something has made it harder or easier for things to pass in and out of the protective cell membrane. Injury could also mean an increase in the amount of lipid or fat in the blood. If a cell is "injured," it could respond by taking defensive steps that might trigger the initiation of a plaque. Inter-estingly enough, cigarette smokers develop different types of plaque lesions than nonsmokers, which suggests that something in tobacco may also cause injury to the endothelium of certain arteries.

The second theory, known as the monoclonal hypothesis, likens plaque to a benign tumor that forms when a single muscle cell from the media travels to the intima and starts wildly multiplying, similar to the uncontrolled growth of cancer cells. People who support this theory believe that the troublesome cell is transformed by some kind of mutagen, perhaps a chemical or a virus that activates or alters a gene so that it behaves differently.

Both theories are intelligent and imaginative, and highlight the importance of understanding the mechanisms of disease at the cellular level. In fact, some researchers believe that one day we will be able to halt arteriosclerosis by developing drugs that will stop the process in its earliest stages. Wouldn't it be wonderful if we could treat this disease long before arteries become clogged with plaque, sparing millions of people the anguish of heart attack and stroke!

WHAT IS CHOLESTEROL?

Despite the bad press cholesterol is getting these days, human beings cannot live without it. Cholesterol is a waxy, yellowish, fatlike substance that is produced in the liver—a virtual cholesterol factory—and in lesser amounts in the intestines and specialized cells throughout the tissues. It is also found in certain foods, mainly dairy products or animal fats.

Cholesterol does some very important things in the body. It is essential for the production of cell membranes. It is a critical ingredient in the making of sex hormones including estrogen. It is needed to produce vitamin D (which is necessary for calcium metabolism), bile (which is used to absorb fat from the intestines), and myelin (the fatty coat that surrounds nerves).

Cholesterol is found in breast milk and added to commercial formula because it is essential for the normal growth and development of infants. After the first year of life, however, our body is capable of producing all the cholesterol we need. So even if we don't consume a single spoonful of cholesterol from outside sources, we would be able to manufacture the 1,000 or so milligrams a day we need to keep us running efficiently. In most cases, the more cholesterol we get from our food, the less we produce on our own. However, if we eat a diet high in saturated fat—a type of fat typically found in meat, whole-milk dairy products, and tropical oils—our body will produce more cholesterol.

Whether or not we ingest cholesterol from the foods we eat, or produce it ourselves, it must be metabolized—that is, converted or broken down into a form that can be used by the body. It must be sent to the cells that need it, and the excess must be stored for future use.

Cholesterol is basically a fat. Since fat is essentially an oil, it is not soluble in water, or in blood, because blood is almost entirely water. Therefore, to travel through the blood stream, fat must be carried as part of a complex molecule called a lipoprotein, which is produced by many tissues in the body. Each lipoprotein contains two kinds of fats which are important sources of energy: cholesterol and triglycerides. These ingredients are combined with a protein called an apoprotein, which allows the fat to be successfully mixed with the blood. Lipoproteins are classified according to their size and the proportion of each of the three essential components they contain.

When we eat fat, chylomicrons, or miniature fat molecules, are formed in the wall of the intestine. These are the largest of all the lipoproteins. They pass into vessels draining the intestine called the lymphatics. From the lymphatic system, the chylomicrons are discharged into our veins and begin their travels through the bloodstream. In the process, various agents work on them to decrease their size, gradually converting chylomicrons into lipids called triglycerides. Most of these are deposited in fatty tissues throughout the body, but some are broken up still further and delivered to the liver, an important factory for processing lipids. In rare cases, what is left of the chylomicron is not delivered to the liver and is allowed to remain in the bloodstream. When this happens, the patient is said to have a disorder called hyperlipidemia that usually requires treatment by medication, a special diet, or both.

In a series of complicated steps, the liver repackages the fats within the now-much-smaller chylomicron into low-density lipids, or LDL, popularly known as the "bad" cholesterol. Some of this cholesterol is delivered to tissues for cell membrane production, repair, and the manufacture of necessary hormones in the body. Some of the LDL is changed still further and transformed into the so-called high-density lipids, or HDL, known as the "good" cholesterol, allowing for excess cholesterol to be secreted back into the intestine so that it can be eliminated from the body.

LDL is the body's major carrier of cholesterol and is believed to be a leading culprit in the formation of plaque. Cells have special receptors or binders on their surfaces that latch on to LDLs, pulling them through the cell membrane into the cell, where they are used to repair old cells and to produce new ones. When the cells have enough cholesterol to do their work, however, they stop producing receptors, allowing the LDL to remain in the blood. Researchers believe that high levels of LDL in blood can actually injure the innermost layer of the artery wall—the endothelium—thus triggering the production of plaque. It is also believed that some people may be born with a genetic inability to produce enough receptors for LDL, resulting in abnormally high levels of this lipoprotein in the blood.

If LDL is the villain of this story, HDL is the heroine. HDL has a very important job. It carries the unused cholesterol to the liver for secretion in the bile. The bile empties into the intestine, flushing excess cholesterol out of the body.

When a laboratory measures total blood cholesterol, it is actually measuring the amount of cholesterol found in one deciliter of blood. Through further testing, the total cholesterol can be broken down into its components: The most important of these are LDL, HDL, and triglyceride. A substantially higher than normal level of any lipid other than HDL (the good fat) is a sign of hyperlipidemia, a condition believed to increase greatly the risk for CAD and even some forms of cancer including colon cancer and breast cancer. Forms of hyperlipidemia may be genetic, or may be a result of a high-fat diet, or both.

RESEARCH

Although physicians have been aware of CAD and arteriosclerosis for centuries, it wasn't until the past few decades that they drew the connection between cholesterol and clogged arteries. They also knew that people who died of heart attacks often had coronary arteries that were filled with plaque, and that there was a probable connection between the incidence of plaque and angina. However, scientists could only speculate on why some people and not others developed plaque in the coronary arteries, and at what age these mysterious lesions began to appear.

In 1915, Sahykov, a Russian scientist, made a startling discovery. He documented evidence of early arteriosclerotic changes in the aortas of children, the large artery that receives the blood from the left ventricle of the heart and distributes it to the body. Today, we call these changes fatty streaks. From then on, scientists speculated that arteriosclerosis was a progressive disease that somehow worsened with age.

Many questions still remained unanswered. What exactly caused those mysterious lesions in some arteries? What was the significance of these fatty streaks in children? Were these fatty streaks the precursors of arteriosclerosis? And finally, why was heart attack the number one killer in the United States, with more and more cases being reported each year?

Researchers were puzzled by the fact that Americans and Western Europeans were especially vulnerable to CAD, but in countries like Japan and Greece, it was a rare disease. Was there anything that we were doing wrong that might be causing this epidemic—or was there anything that they were doing right that could prevent it? Dietary habits seemed to be the most striking and consistent difference. Americans and Western Europeans—devotees of the meat and potato cuisines—ate diets high in saturated fat and cholesterol, on average consuming between 40 percent and 50 percent of their total daily calories in the form of fat. People in countries with the lowest rates of heart disease ate low-fat diets consisting mainly of fish, grains, and vegetables, on average consuming less than 25 percent of their total daily calories in the form of fat.

A study of nineteen countries by the World Health Organization showed a direct relationship between the intake of dietary fat and cholesterol and the incidence of CAD. In sum, countries that consumed the highest amount of saturated fat in their diet had on average the highest cholesterol levels—typically above 250 mg/dl—and the highest rate of CAD. Countries that consumed the least amount of saturated fat had the lowest cholesterol levels—typically below 150 mg/dl—and the lowest rate of CAD.

Skeptics still questioned whether the culprit was genetics rather than diet.

Could it be that some populations were genetically prone to develop arteriosclerosis, whereas others were born with an immunity against arterial damage? The Japan–Honolulu–San Francisco study begun in 1965 shed some light on this controversy. In this study, researchers observed the eating habits of three groups of Japanese men. The first group were native Japanese who lived in Japan, who ate the traditional low-fat, low-cholesterol diet—lots of rice, sushi, and seaweed. The second group were native Japanese who had moved to Hawaii, and as a result, were now eating a diet richer in saturated fat and cholesterol. And the third group were native Japanese who had moved to San Francisco, and were eating a typical American diet high in saturated fat and cholesterol.

In a follow-up study ten years later, researchers showed that the men who had remained in Japan had the lowest cholesterol and lowest rate of heart disease. Those who had moved to Honolulu had higher cholesterol levels than those who had stayed in Japan, and proportionally higher rates of heart disease. And those who had moved to San Francisco—where they were presumably gorging on cheeseburgers and fries like the rest of us—had the highest cholesterol levels and the highest rate of heart disease.

Animal studies also confirm the theory that a diet laden with fat can promote heart disease. For years, scientists have been able to induce arteriosclerosis in the coronary arteries of animals such as geese and swine by feeding them a diet rich in saturated fats. When the same animals were fed a low-fat diet, the arteries slowly opened, although some blockage remained.

Until very recently, however, it's been extremely difficult to prove that arteriosclerosis can be reversed in humans at all. A handful of small, carefully designed studies have shown that people with CAD can partially reopen their coronary arteries if they drastically change their diet and lifestyle, but as of this writing, no single study has shown that dietary changes alone can produce this kind of improvement, or that people who adopt low-fat diets to lower their cholesterol levels live any longer than those who don't.

In 1990—nearly two decades after the cholesterol controversy began—a ground-breaking study finally offered conclusive proof that in some cases a significant reduction in cholesterol can save lives. The Program on the Surgical Control of the Hyperlipidemias (POSCH) followed 838 patients (90 percent were men) who had survived heart attacks for more than ten years. Out of that group, 421 underwent a surgical procedure called partial ileal bypass in which a portion of the intestine was removed, thus resulting in an average 20 percent reduction in blood cholesterol levels. The rest of the patients were treated with cholesterol-lowering drugs that reduced their cholesterol levels by only 10 percent on average.

The study showed that those who had the surgery and experienced the 20 percent reduction in cholesterol fared far better than those who did not. The surgery subjects showed a slower progression of arteriosclerosis and were less likely to have another heart attack that those who only took the cholesterol-lowering drugs. In addition, the study revealed that surgery patients who still had a well-functioning heart after their heart attack were less likely to die than patients with good heart function who did not have surgery (24 out of 281 of the surgery group with good heart function died, versus 39 out of 292 of the nonsurgery group).

This finding is very significant because for the first time researchers drew a positive link between lowering cholesterol and reducing mortality. Although the surgical procedure appears to save lives, it is not without discomfort or risk. Many patients had chronic diarrhea after the surgery, while others developed gallstones, kidney stones, and intestinal obstructions. As impressive as the results of this study may be, it is unlikely that this procedure will be widely used as a means of reducing cholesterol.

Other studies designed to investigate the cholesterol–heart disease link—specifically looking at whether lowering cholesterol would reduce the risk of CAD—have yielded interesting results. Even though these major studies have excluded women, I believe that their findings are still relevant. One of the most famous studies is the Coronary Primary Prevention Trial reported in 1984, which involved 3,806 men between the ages of thirty-five and sixty-nine who had no evidence of CAD. The men in the study all had cholesterol levels higher than 265 mg/dl. The average cholesterol was 291 mg/dl with average LDLs of 170 mg/dl, which is considered high.

One-half of the participants were given cholestyramine, a special drug designed to lower cholesterol. The other group received a placebo. Because of the unpleasant side effects associated with this drug, including nausea, heart-burn, and bloating, most took a smaller than normal dose. The group on the drug achieved a 9 percent lowering of their cholesterol and cut their rate of heart attack by 19 percent.

From this study, researchers developed the rule of thumb that a 1 percent reduction in cholesterol produces a 2 percent decrease in the risk of developing CAD. Unfortunately, this study did not show that men who took the medication lived any longer than those who did not. In fact, the mortality results were rather bizarre. For some unknown reason, probably unrelated to the study, although these men had fewer fatal heart attacks, they were more prone to die violently or in accidents. Nevertheless, many members of the medical community believe that this study validates the connection between cholesterol and heart disease, at least for men.

Another often-quoted study involving men is the Oslo Study Diet and Antismoking Trial. The well-known study followed 1,232 men: Half of them were nonsmokers (who formerly smoked) on low-fat, low-cholesterol diets and the other half were smokers on typically high-fat diets. By the end of a five-year period, cholesterol levels for the group on the special diet had been reduced by an average of 13 percent, compared with only 3 percent in the other group. The group with the lower cholesterol had a 47 percent lower rate of CAD, including fatal and nonfatal heart attacks.

Follow-up studies continue to show that the participants who ate the low-fat diet have lower rates of CAD and mortality. Because the men in the study on a low-fat diet had also stopped smoking, it is difficult to tell whether diet alone was responsible for the drop in cholesterol, or the incidence of CAD. However, I feel that this study provides a valuable lesson for both men and women: If you want to reduce your chances of CAD, work on lowering your cholesterol to safe levels and don't smoke.

Based on studies that showed a correlation between cholesterol and heart disease, in the mid-1980s, the American Heart Association and the federal government joined forces to create the National Cholesterol Education Program (NCEP). Their goal is to convince Americans that the average cholesterol level of 220–240 mg/dl is too high. According to the NCEP:

· Cholesterol levels of 200 mg/dl or less are desirable.
· People with cholesterol levels between 200 mg/dl and 239 mg/dl are considered at "moderate high risk," but they are not advised to take any measures to lower their cholesterol unless they have two or more other risk factors for CAD.
· People with cholesterol levels above 240 mg/dl are considered to be at high risk and are advised to work with their physicians to lower their cholesterol to a safer level.

The NCEP also recommends that Americans restrict their intake of fat to less than 30 percent of their daily total calories, with no more than 10 percent coming from saturated fat. If moderate dietary change does not lower elevated cholesterol within six months, or if patients are at extremely high risk, the NCEP advises physicians to put these patients on an even more stringent diet of no more than 7 percent saturated fat, and to consider using a cholesterol-lowering medication.

It may be decades before the diet–cholesterol–heart disease controversy is resolved and a definitive study finally lays all these doubts to rest. Does that mean that we should eat, drink, and be merry until everyone in the medical community agrees on the causes of arteriosclerosis? Of course not.

Although some of the studies may be flawed, I believe it would be a terrible mistake to ignore the important information that they have to offer—information that could help save our lives and the lives of loved ones. It would also be downright foolish to ignore the handful of studies that do include women, which more often than not concur with the studies that exclude them. Below are some of the major studies that have investigated the causes of arteriosclerosis and have included women.

Framingham Study

It may not be a top tourist attraction, but Framingham, Massachusetts, will have a special place in the history books. For more than forty years, the Framingham study of the National Heart, Lung and Blood Institute has followed the progress of 2,336 men and 2,873 women, ages thirty to sixty-three, all residents of this small New England town, to study the causes, risk factors, and course of CAD. One of the study's most important features is that it has followed the same subjects for a very long time period. Most other work has been done for much shorter periods.

Because Framingham is one of the few major studies to include women, it has become an invaluable source of information for those of us who are concerned about women's health. From Framingham we learned a number of startling facts. For example, although we knew that there was a connection between diabetes and heart disease, we didn't know how serious it was until Framingham proved that women with diabetes ran the same risk of heart disease as men, regardless of age.

Framingham was also the first study to show a direct correlation between elevated cholesterol and heart disease for both men and women (although it did not show a connection between diet and cholesterol). There is not enough room in this chapter to list all the things that we have learned from Framingham. This study has spawned scores of research articles. It has provided us with a wealth of information about the possible causes of CAD. And it has given us important information directly related to women:

· Until age fifty, increasing levels of serum cholesterol directly correlate to the incidence of CAD. In other words, women with the highest overall cholesterol are the ones most likely to develop heart disease.
· At any age, women with the highest cholesterol levels are the ones most likely to suffer strokes.
· After age fifty, there is no direct correlation between the level of serum cholesterol and the incidence of CAD. However, women with the lowest levels of HDL have the highest rates of CAD. Even a small reduction in HDL greatly increases the risk of heart disease.
· The ratio between total cholesterol and HDL should not exceed 6:1. For example, if the total cholesterol is 240, HDL should be 40 or more. A higher than 6:1 ratio increases a woman's risk of CAD. The HDL:LDL

ratio ideally should be 3:1 or better, but should not exceed 4:1. Therefore if the LDL is 120, the HDL should be 40 or more.

· Elevated triglyceride levels—higher than 190 mg/dl—are the best predictor of coronary artery disease in women, but not in men. High triglyceride levels are particularly dangerous to women. Levels higher than 400 mg/dl are dangerous to both sexes.

· Women with elevated LDL levels—higher than 130 mg/dl—have only a slightly higher risk of developing CAD than those with normal levels. In other words, although high LDL is not good for either sex, they do not appear to be as devastating for women as they are for men.

· For women, dramatic increases in the rate of CAD occurred at cholesterol levels of 265 mg/dl and higher, which is considerably higher than the 240 mg/dl usually cited for men. This finding doesn't mean that it's safe to allow your cholesterol to go up this high, especially if you have other risk factors. But it does suggest that women may tolerate higher levels of cholesterol than men, probably because a greater portion of their cholesterol is in the form of beneficial HDL. Thus, the total blood cholesterol level for women can be misleading if it is the only figure being used to determine risk for CAD. For example, if a woman has a cholesterol of 245 and an HDL of 85, she would still be considered at relatively low risk for CAD. However, that same 245 cholesterol would be considered high risk if her HDL was below 40.

These are just some of the facts that we've learned from the Framingham study, a national treasure that has saved the lives of countless numbers of Americans. As you can see, although overall cholesterol level is important, it does not provide enough information. It is also important for women to know their levels of HDL and triglyceride. Therefore, I recommend that all of my patients have a complete lipid profile taken at their first examination. If the profile is completely normal, I do a follow-up annually. If there's a problem, I retest more frequently.

Lipid Research Clinics Follow-up Study

This study examined risk factors for CAD in 2,000 women between the ages of forty and sixty-nine, in ten different clinics throughout the country from 1972 to 1976. As had the Framingham study, this work showed that women with elevated LDL were only slightly more likely to develop CAD than those with normal levels. But it also revealed that a 10 mg/dl reduction in HDL increases a woman's risk of heart disease by 50 percent! Once again, this study confirmed the belief that low HDL is a more accurate predictor of heart disease for women than high LDL. This study also found that when cholesterol levels rose to 235 mg/dl, the risk of death due to CAD increased 70 percent.

Nurses' Health Study

In 1976, 121,700 married female registered nurses filled out questionnaires designed to discover the major risk factors for women for CAD. The nurses were asked a wide variety of questions about their health, including whether or not they were under treatment for high cholesterol or any other condition that could contribute to the onset of CAD. This study, which is periodically updated, shows that women with elevated cholesterol levels are twice as likely to develop CAD than those with normal levels.

Rancho Bernardo

The ten-year study included 2,048 women in this southern California planned community between the ages of fifty and seventy-nine. Researchers found that women with cholesterol levels higher than 260 mg/dl had a 2.5 times increased risk of developing CAD. Once again, women with the highest rates of cholesterol were more likely to die from a heart attack than those with lower levels.

IMPORTANCE OF CHOLESTEROL TESTS

What have we learned from these studies? Low levels of HDL cholesterol and/or elevated triglycerides are dangerous for women and are strong predictors of CAD. To a lesser extent, elevated total blood cholesterol and high LDLs are also risk factors for CAD. For women, total cholesterol is also an important risk factor for stroke, and certainly should not be ignored. Women need and should have this information.

There are several methods of testing the blood for an elevated level of fat. A simple cholesterol screening that can be done almost anywhere is less complex than an extensive lipid profile that can be analyzed only at a special laboratory. Since simple cholesterol screening tests are cheap and easy to perform, they are done more frequently. In my opinion, an isolated serum cholesterol reading is not useful. Such a test does not give necessary information about other blood lipids. It does not assess HDL or triglycerides. As for mass screening programs for high cholesterol, there have been distressing news reports citing unsanitary conditions, poorly trained staff, and faulty testing equipment. I feel your best bet is to have a lipid test performed in your doctor's office where a tested commercial laboratory will be reporting the results and your doctor will be on hand to interpret and fully explain the numbers to you.

I believe that every woman should have a complete lipid profile taken by her thirtieth birthday and certainly before menopause. Unless there is a problem, she need not have the test redone until the following year. If her HDL is low, or her triglycerides are high, she will require close monitoring and advice about her diet, stress levels, exercise programs, and possibly weight loss. She should also be told if she has additional risk factors for developing CAD. Finally, women who plan to start and continue the use of oral contraceptives should have their lipid profile tested annually. Women who have a primary relative— parent, sibling, or grandparent—with hyperlipidemia should have a lipid profile done before age eighteen.

A word of caution: Even the best laboratory can make mistakes. Some experts estimate that there can be as much as a 30-point variation in cholesterol levels depending on the laboratory and the type of machinery used. It's important to know, therefore, that one abnormal value for any serum lipid level should not lead to decisions about therapy. In my practice a minimum of three abnormal values in a patient fasting for at least 12 hours, taken at similar times in the day and tested by the same laboratory, are necessary before I decide to treat the disorder. If over time a patient has shown consistently abnormal values, I accept the numbers. On the other hand, if a report comes back that indicates a previously undetected problem, I don't hesitate to repeat the test as a precaution against treating a patient unnecessarily. I do the same thing if I get a test result that is radically different from a previous one.

What if I find out that someone has a dangerously high cholesterol or triglyceride level? If the patient is obese, weight loss is essential; this, combined with changes in the diet and a regular exercise program, corrects the problem in many patients. Some patients, however, are unable to lose weight and are unwilling to exercise. When all efforts fail, I feel that it is appropriate to discuss drug therapy with the patient, especially if she has other risk factors for developing arteriosclerosis. There is no rule of thumb here. Each patient must be carefully evaluated and each must understand the risks and benefits of therapy before she agrees to it. The first step should be a thorough blood and urine analysis. The decision to treat a high cholesterol or high triglyceride level is not an easy one. To show just how complicated it can be, see the three patient profiles starting on page 68.

LAB REPORT
BLOOD AND URINE ANALYSIS

TEST	RESULT	OUT OF RANGE (OR INTERPRETATION)	UNITS	REFERENCE RANGE	SC
CARE 1 PANEL					
CHEMZYME					NY
ALKALINE PHOSPHATASE	56		U/L	20 - 140	
LACTIC DEHYDROGENASE	175		U/L	0-250	
SGO-TRANSAMINASE	23		U/L	0-50	
SGP-TRANSAMINASE	26		U/L	0-55	
BILIRUBIN, TOTAL	0.6		MG/DL	0.2-1.2	
PROTEIN, TOTAL	7.3		GM/DL	6.0-8.5	
ALBUMIN	4.4		GM/DL	3.2-5.5	
SODIUM	141		MEQ/L	135-148	
POTASSIUM	4.5		MEQ/L	3.5-5.3	
CHLORIDE	100		MEQ/L	95-110	
CARBON DIOXIDE CONTENT	25		MEQ/L	20-34	
CALCIUM	9.2		MG/DL	8.5-10.6	
PHOSPHOROUS, INORGANIC	3.8		MG/DL	2.5-4.5	
GLUCOSE	83		MG/DL	70-115	
CREATININE	1.2		MG/DL	0.7-1.4	
UREA NITROGEN	16		MG/DL	7-25	
URIC ACID	5.0		MG/DL	4.0-8.5	
GLOBULIN	2.9		GM/DL	1.5-3.8	
A/G RATIO	1.5			1.01/1-2.20/1	
BUN/CREATININE RATIO	13.3			8.0-20.0	
TRIGLYCERIDES		185 H	MG/DL	20-160	
CHOLESTEROL, TOTAL		211 H	MG/DL		

```
                    ADULT REFERENCE RANGE
       LESS THAN 200 MG/DL - DESIRABLE SERUM CHOLESTEROL
              200-239 MG/DL - BORDERLINE HIGH CHOLESTEROL
       GREATER THAN 240 MG/DL - HIGH SERUM CHOLESTEROL
```

IRON, TOTAL	75		MCG/DL	55-185	
LIPID RATIO CALCULATIONS					NY
HDL CHOLESTEROL		32 L	MG/DL		

REFERENCE RANGE	RISK LEVEL
----------------	----------
LESS THAN 45 MG/DL:	INCREASED
45 MG/DL:	AVERAGE
GREATER THAN 45 MG/DL:	DECREASED

>> REPORT CONTINUED ON NEXT PAGE <<

TEST	RESULT	OUT OF RANGE (OR INTERPRETATION)	UNITS	REFERENCE RANGE	SC

LIPID RATIO CALCULATIONS (CONTINUED)

| LDL CHOLESTEROL | | 142 H | MG/DL | | |

REFERENCE RANGE: LESS THAN 130 MG/DL

THE LDL CHOLESTEROL IS A CALCULATED RESULT BASED ON
THE CHOLESTEROL, TRIGLYCERIDE AND HDL CHOLESTEROL
CONCENTRATIONS.

CHOLESTEROL/HDL RATIO   6.6

REFERENCE RANGE
INTERPRETATION OF CHOLESTEROL / HDL RATIO

RISK	CHOL/HDL (FEMALE)	CHOL/HDL (MALE)
1/2 AVERAGE	3.27	3.43
AVERAGE	4.44	4.97
2X AVERAGE	7.05	9.50
3X AVERAGE	11.04	23.99

CBC WITH DIFF + PLATELET   NY

TEST	RESULT	OUT OF RANGE	UNITS	REFERENCE RANGE
WHITE BLOOD CELLS		11.9 H	THOUS/CUMM	3.8-10.1
RED BLOOD CELLS	5.46		MIL/CUMM	4.40-5.80
HEMOGLOBIN	15.8		G/DL	13.8-17.2
HEMATOCRIT	47.4		%	41.0-50.0
MCV	86.9		CU MICRONS	80.0-100.0
MCH	28.9		PG	27.0-33.0
MCHC	33.3		%	32.0-36.0
NEUTROPHILS	72		%	40-75
LYMPHOCYTES	20		%	18-47
MONOCYTES	5		%	0-10
EOSINOPHILS	3		%	0-6
BASOPHILS	0		%	0-2
PLATELET COUNT	224		THOUS/CUMM	130-400

URINALYSIS   NY

TEST	RESULT	REFERENCE RANGE
COLOR	YELLOW	YELLOW
APPEARANCE	CLEAR	CLEAR
SPECIFIC GRAVITY	1.025	1.001-1.035
PH (REACTION)	5.0	4.6-8.0
GLUCOSE QUALITATIVE	NEGATIVE	NEGATIVE
PROTEIN QUALITATIVE	NEGATIVE	NEGATIVE

>> REPORT CONTINUED ON NEXT PAGE <<

TEST	RESULT	OUT OF RANGE (OR INTERPRETATION)	UNITS	REFERENCE RANGE	SC
URINALYSIS (CONTINUED)					
ACETONE QUALITATIVE	NEGATIVE			NEGATIVE	
OCCULT BLOOD	NEGATIVE			NEGATIVE	
BILE QUALITATIVE	NEGATIVE			NEGATIVE	
NITRITE	NEGATIVE			NEGATIVE	
LEUKOCYTE ESTERASE	NEGATIVE			NEGATIVE	
WBC	0-1			0-5/HPF	
SQUAMOUS EPITHELIAL CELLS	FEW			FEW	
SED RATE WESTERGREN	1		MM/HR	0-15	NY
RPR	NON-REACTIVE			NON-REACTIVE	NY

>> END OF REPORT <<

CASE HISTORY 1
ROSE L.

LIPID PROFILE
CHOLESTEROL 310
HDL 45
TRIGLYCERIDES 250

In every doctor's caseload, there are one or two patients who are more of a concern than others. Rose, an energetic seventy-five-year-old retired teacher, was one of those worrisome people. Rose was doing everything right: She exercised regularly, ate a low-fat diet, and religiously kept her appointments with me. In spite of her healthy lifestyle, her cholesterol was 310 mg/dl and seemed to be edging upward each year. Her blood pressure was also high. Despite the fact that older people have higher cholesterol levels than their younger counterparts, these levels, which we confirmed three times in a fasting state, were beginning to be a concern.

Although a mild diuretic controlled her blood pressure quite well most of the time, whenever she was upset or anxious, the reading soared. During her last office visit, Rose complained of occasional dizziness. Much to my distress, I noticed that the normally quick-witted, fast-talking New Yorker seemed to be irritable and confused. I was very worried.

With high blood pressure and high cholesterol, Rose was a prime candidate for a stroke. In fact, I believed that the dizzy spells she spoke of were actually transient ischemic attacks (TIAs): ministrokes that usually precede a bigger and more debilitating stroke. To reduce her risk, Rose's blood pressure and cholesterol had to be lowered to safer levels. Since she was already on a low-fat diet, Rose would require medication. But choosing the right medicine to treat high cholesterol requires careful thought and discussion of the options with the patient. Under the best of circumstances, these drugs can cause unpleasant if not serious side effects, ranging from nausea to liver damage. To further complicate matters, Rose was highly allergic and often had adverse reactions to the mildest of medications. In her case, I had to be very careful about selecting the drug I felt would have the fewest side effects.

My first thought was the newest cholesterol-lowering drug, lovastatin, which is a lot more pleasant to take than some of the older ones. But it wasn't the best choice for Rose. Studies suggest that the drug might increase the incidence of cataracts. Since Rose already had one cataract in each eye, lovastatin was out of the question.

I next thought about nicotinic acid, which is extremely effective, but can cause flushing in many patients and may cause very dry, itchy skin or even a troublesome rash. Of course, I could write a prescription for ibuprofen to alleviate the flushing, but I preferred that Rose take only one drug, not two. I spent days thinking about how to solve the problem.

I finally decided, after explaining all of the options to my patient, to try cholestyramine, warning her that she might have to deal with two annoying side effects: increased constipation and possible nausea or flatulence. Well aware of the dangers of allowing her cholesterol to remain high, Rose agreed to take the drug. I started her on a very low dose, moving up gradually and monitoring her cholesterol to make sure she was on the lowest possible dose to produce the desired effect.

Rose's cholesterol is now down to 255, which has improved her HDL-to-total-cholesterol ratio and her triglycerides are a safer 170. Despite the initial discomfort involved in taking this medication, I believe that Rose is now much better protected against the possibility of having a debilitating stroke.

CASE HISTORY 2
GAIL R.

LIPID PROFILE
CHOLESTEROL 289
HDL 40
TRIGLYCERIDE 300

Gail is another example of a woman with high cholesterol who needed treatment, but not just because of the cholesterol. At forty-eight years old with high blood pressure, Gail was entering menopause 30 pounds overweight, with a cholesterol of 289 mg/dl and extremely high triglycerides. (I had tested these values several times, warning Gail not to drink any alcohol for 48 hours before I did so. Alcohol can temporarily raise triglycerides to three times a patient's usual level.) Gail has been on two drugs for high blood pressure for five years.

Gail's sedentary lifestyle is in part responsible for her health problems. Behind a desk all day at work, her evening recreation usually consists of cooking or eating out with her husband after an extended cocktail hour. When I suggested that she lose some weight, she laughed. When I suggested she take up walking or some other form of moderate exercise, she simply tuned me out. I've known Gail for years, and I realize that no matter how strong a case I try to make, she will never trade in her copies of *Gourmet* for *Prevention*. It is just not her style. After trying several times to enlist her collaboration in a plan to change some of the interests and habits I felt were hurting her, I realized that continuing on this path would alienate her and make her defensive and guilty when she came to see me. Together, we acknowledged that the final choices were hers and that my job was to help her reduce her risk factors in a manner she could live with.

Since I believe that Gail is at serious risk of having a heart attack or stroke, I felt I had no choice but to prescribe lovastatin despite the fact that I thought it was only the second-best solution. However, I felt very strongly that not treating her might well have condemned her to a life of disability or even premature death. On the drug, her cholesterol dropped to 220. Her triglycerides are now 210. I haven't given up on Gail. From time to time, I try again to help her find other ways to help her enjoy her leisure time; I have even suggested to her husband, who loves her dearly, that the ideal solution might be to find a sport that they could do together. So far, however, the restaurants are winning.

CASE HISTORY 3
HELEN G.

LIPID PROFILE
CHOLESTEROL 260
HDL 80
TRIGLYCERIDE 150

Finally, I'm going to tell you about a patient that I decided not to treat even though her cholesterol was about 260 mg/dl. Her HDLs were high at 80 and her triglycerides were excellent. Helen, a fifty-three-year-old advertising executive, dons Reeboks every morning and walks to work. A trim 125 pounds, she eats sensibly, goes to an aerobics class twice a week, and gets a lot of pleasure out of her interesting life. She has many friends, and at least once a week she supplements her diversified and engrossing work with concerts or the theater. Her parents lived to be well in their eighties.

I am treating Helen for a congenital heart condition that has nothing to do with CAD. Do I put a woman like Helen on a very restrictive diet or on medication to lower her cholesterol? No. Instead I recommended that Helen meet with a nutritionist with whom I work to see if there were some easy ways for her to reduce fat in her diet without having to change drastically her eating style. But other than that, I recheck her serum lipids every year just to make sure they aren't getting any higher. I expect that Helen will follow in her parents' footsteps and live a long and healthy life.

EFFECTIVE TREATMENT PROGRAMS

As you can see from these stories, numbers alone don't tell the whole story: An effective treatment program involves an assessment of every patient as a person. The good doctor considers the family history, whether or not other risk factors are present, and whether or not she can convince the patient that changing her lifestyle is both worthwhile and doable. No patient should ever be bullied or made to feel uncomfortable because a healthy lifestyle seems less important than giving up the pleasures that may be tremendously comforting to her. Finally, the doctor must not overreact: An otherwise perfectly healthy woman with no risk factors should not be thrown into a panic over an elevated cholesterol level. However, a woman with other risk factors such as obesity, smoking, or hypertension must take a high cholesterol level very seriously. In fact, she may even need to keep the level lower than average to avert a disaster.

In most physicians' minds, the first step in treating high cholesterol is dietary modification and exercise. Through changes in eating patterns, patients are often able to reduce their cholesterol by anywhere from 10 percent to 20 percent. I often have my patients see a nutritionist who helps them devise a diet plan they can live with. In my experience, it is not enough to hand a patient a sheet of paper with dietary guidelines and expect them to follow it on their own. Within a few weeks, those papers usually end up at the bottom of a desk drawer or even in the garbage can. Changing a lifetime of bad eating habits requires education, special tailoring to the individual's tastes and cultural background, follow-up, and continual support. In chapter 19 I discuss nutrition.

Exercise is an essential component of the treatment plan. Several studies have shown that exercise can lower cholesterol and raise HDL in women. In fact, according to one recent study, even the mildest forms of exercise, such as a half-hour brisk walk two or three times a week, can significantly reduce the risk of CAD and stroke. It can also help you look and feel terrific.

If diet and exercise alone can't reduce cholesterol to within "safe" limits, your doctor may have to prescribe one of several cholesterol-lowering drugs. We don't like to prescribe these drugs indiscriminately for several reasons: First, they all have side effects that at best cause the patient temporary discomfort, and at worst, they could be dangerous. Second, once you're on them, you have to stay on them for a lifetime; they aren't a cure, and if you stop the drug, the serum lipids go right back up. Finally, they're expensive. They can cost thousands of dollars a year.

Despite the risks and the expense, I am convinced that in some cases these medications have helped save the lives of my patients or spared them from debilitating cardiovascular illness. Needless to say, anyone starting to take a cholesterol-lowering drug should be carefully monitored by her physician. When I begin a patient on this type of medication, I call her frequently to make sure that the dose is appropriate and the patient is not experiencing any unusual reactions. Visits to the doctor at least every two weeks are a good idea, with monitoring of the lipid response to the therapy at each visit. A lipid check every three months is enough once the condition is stabilized. See page 72 for a list of drugs commonly used to lower cholesterol.

I've said repeatedly throughout this chapter that I will prescribe medication for high cholesterol only in cases where other risk factors are present, and when all other nonmedical solutions have failed. It's important to remember that although high cholesterol is an important risk factor for CAD, it is not the only one. High blood pressure, smoking, family medical history, and even stress are also important risk factors that need to be considered each time we counsel a patient.

As we end the twentieth century, we know a great deal more about CAD than we did when we began it. But it may be well into the twenty-first century before we have a complete understanding of the disease process, and more importantly, of how to prevent it.

DRUGS USED FOR THE TREATMENT OF HIGH CHOLESTEROL

Drug	Trade Name	How It Works	Some Side Effects
BILE ACID SEQUESTRANTS			
Cholestyramine Colestipol	Questran Colestid	Binds bile acids in the intestine so they are eliminated from the body rather than reabsorbed	Gastrointestinal discomfort such as constipation; can interfere with vitamin absorption and therefore should not be taken during pregnancy
Niacin (Nicotinic acid)	Nia-Bid	Mechanism unknown; lowers LDL and can increase HDL	Flushing of skin, itching of skin, skin rash; nausea; liver damage; effects on fetus not studied
FIBRIC ACID DERIVATIVES			
Clofibrate Gemfibrozil	Atromid-S Lopid	Exact mechanism unknown; lowers LDL, but can also increase HDL	Gastrointestinal distress; gallstones; headache; fatigue; muscle cramps; effects on fetus not studied
Lovastatin	Mevacor	Retards synthesis of cholesterol; lowers LDL	Liver damage; may increase cataracts; can be dangerous to combine with some other cholesterol-lowering drugs
Probucol	Lorelco	Increases rate of breakdown of LDL	Gastrointestinal distress, including gas, nausea, and diarrhea; can produce cardiac arrhythmia

Adapted from information in *Medical Letter:* 30:81–84, 1988.

Chapter 6

ANGINA

It felt as if someone had put a belt around my chest and was squeezing it tighter and tighter.

All I felt was pain in my left arm. I thought I had pulled a muscle.

It felt as if my chest was on fire and then it went away.

—Three women describing an angina attack

ANGINA, a term derived from Greek, meaning "to strangle," is a condition that occurs when the heart is not getting enough oxygen, usually due to arteriosclerosis or a temporary narrowing of a coronary artery due to spasm. Women are reported to have a higher incidence of angina and angina-like pain than men. In 56 percent of cases of women with CAD, angina or chest pain is the first warning sign. Often, a heart supplied by partially obstructed or narrowed coronaries functions quite well until something happens that suddenly increases the demand for cardiac work. For example, a previously sedentary person may begin an exercise program that places an added burden on her heart. Because of the underlying arterial disease, blood flow cannot increase to carry enough oxygen to the working muscle and the pain of oxygen deprivation is felt for the first time.

Angina is not a heart attack in which portions of heart muscle are rendered useless forever. Once the angina passes and blood is restored to the deprived area—usually in less than a minute—the heart cells function quite normally. This is not to say that angina is a minor symptom. In fact, in some cases, it means a full-blown heart attack is occurring or it is a precursor of a heart attack soon to come. However, in 80 percent of all cases of angina involving women, the pain passes and does not develop into a heart attack.

SYMPTOMS AND DIAGNOSIS

Angina means different things to different people. Some people experience classic angina—a heaviness, burning, or squeezing in the chest, often radiating to the back, up to the neck, and sometimes down the left arm. However, not all angina conforms to this textbook definition. In fact, the variations of angina can often be very confusing. For example, I recently saw a forty-nine-year-old woman who had for several years complained of chronic pain in her jaw. In fact, her dentist had already pulled out three of her teeth in the belief that the pain was a result of their decay. Yet the pain persisted and her family doctor finally referred her to me.

After taking a complete history and listening—not just nodding and taking notes but really listening—to what this patient had to say, I discovered that the problem had nothing to do with her teeth. She was having angina—not the garden variety angina most people have, but angina all the same. I reached this conclusion based on two things that she said. First, she described the pain in a very specific way: a sharp twinge lasting for only a few minutes at a time. The last time I had a toothache, it was more like a relentless dull ache that went on for days. Second, she said that it seemed to bother her more when she was tired or under stress than when she was relaxed, which is not typical of a toothache but is definitely a characteristic of angina.

A stress test later revealed that this woman indeed had ischemia, or oxygen deprivation, during exercise. She is now being treated with medication that dilates her coronary arteries and she is free of pain. Why did it take so long for this woman to get an accurate diagnosis? I have a nagging suspicion that if she had been a man her doctor would have at least considered the possibility that her persistent problem, in spite of all the dental attention, was in fact angina.

In all fairness, however, angina is not always easy to diagnose because there are many conditions that mimic it. A burning sensation in the chest may indeed be angina, but it can also be heartburn or countless other digestive disorders. A heaviness might be due to asthma or bronchitis. A sharp pain in the elbow or even in a finger could also be referred pain from angina, but then again, it might well be from a bone or muscle injury. In fact, chest pain accompanying mitral valve prolapse, a condition common in women, is often misdiagnosed as CAD. Often, a doctor may have to perform an extensive examination of the esophagus and upper gastrointestinal tract before diagnosing angina. It may include studies of how they function as well as how they look, both under direct vision using a special endoscope and in special X-ray studies.

Anginal symptoms not only vary from person to person but depending on the individual they can be triggered by different activities or irritants. For example, some people are extremely sensitive to cold: A blast of cold air or an icy drink is all it takes to spark an attack. But other people may experience pain only in times of physical and emotional stress. In fact, for some people, specific events seem to trigger angina. A case in point is my patient Liz, a lawyer in her forties who has spent two decades on the fast track. Rarely getting home before 9 P.M., Liz bounces from crisis to crisis and courtroom to courtroom without ever feeling the slightest twinge. On the weekends when her nineteen-year-old daughter Suzy is home from college, however, Liz complains of chest pains. In fact, nine out of ten times when my beeper goes off on a Saturday night, it's because Suzy's back in town. Liz is not unusual. Like so many other mothers—and I put myself in this category—Liz is able to handle the pressure of work with objectivity and even a sense of humor, but when it comes to her child, her emotions sometimes overpower her. And strong emotions can elicit a strong physical response.

When you experience a strong emotional outburst, as you might when worrying about your teenage daughter, your body's sympathetic nervous system fires off a burst of chemicals that constrict the blood vessels, forcing the heart to beat faster and harder. If the vessels bringing blood to the heart become too narrowed, portions of the heart muscle may not get enough oxygen to fuel the extra work, and angina begins.

Anyone who has had angina-like symptoms should be evaluated by her doctor. If the doctor suspects that it's the real thing, she will probably start with an EKG to test for evidence of injury or irregular heart rhythm. It should be followed by an echocardiogram, a picture of the heart generated by sound waves that tells your doctor a great deal about the structure and function of the heart muscle. She may also order an exercise stress test to look for any evidence of ischemia, or oxygen deprivation, which occurs when the heart is forced to work harder than usual. A 24-hour monitoring of the patient's electrocardiogram, called a Holter, is also very useful to uncover episodes of inadequate blood supply to the heart, which may or may not be accompanied by chest pain.

MEDICATION

If the angina is only occasional, the doctor may prescribe oral nitroglycerine to be taken at the onset of an attack. Placed under the tongue, this very effective drug quickly dilates the arteries, allowing blood to flow more freely through the heart. If the patient is plagued with chronic angina, nitroglycerine can be taken in the form of a transdermal (skin) patch, a Band-Aid-like patch worn on the skin that slowly releases the drug over a 24-hour period. The skin patch is useful to prevent an attack, but does not work fast enough to stop an attack already in progress.

If a patient knows that certain events or activities trigger angina, she can take nitroglycerine beforehand to try to ward off the attack. For example, I have one patient whose sex life was being ruined by chest pains. For her, a prophylactic dose of nitroglycerine did the trick and she was able to engage in sexual activity without worrying.

Nitroglycerine can have some unpleasant side effects. Many patients initially experience headaches, some so severe that they want to dispense with the drug altogether. In most cases, the pain can be relieved by aspirin or acetaminophen and over time the headaches disappear. In addition, nitroglycerine can cause a sudden decline in blood pressure in some people, leaving them feeling weak and unsteady. But there's an easy solution to this problem. These patients should take the drug while sitting or resting and should not resume activity until the feeling has passed.

Another group of drugs called beta blockers—designed to decrease the oxygen demand on the heart by blocking the effect of the sympathetic nervous system on the heart muscle—may be used to control angina. These are a very good choice for people who experience angina when they are upset or under emotional duress, but usually not when angina is related to physical exertion. In recent years, calcium channel blockers have joined the arsenal of weapons against angina. These drugs reduce the flow of calcium into the muscle cells in the walls of the coronary arteries, which helps prevent spasm that so often produces anginal pain. Calcium channel blockers are used alone or with beta blockers to prevent angina attacks.

In many cases, angina can be successfully treated with medication and common sense: getting enough rest, avoiding stressful situations if possible, and becoming attuned to your body so you can pick up any early warning signs that an attack may be imminent. However, if the symptoms change, that is, if the incidence of attacks increases, or the angina worsens, call your doctor immediately. In these cases of so-called unstable angina, other treatments including a change in medication, angioplasty, or even bypass surgery may be considered.

SILENT ISCHEMIA

Silent ischemia is really angina without the pain. Similar to a bona fide anginal attack, the heart is temporarily deprived of sufficient oxygen to meet its demands, but because there's no physical sensation, the victim doesn't know it. No one knows why some people have pain and others don't. In fact, no one knows the actual cause of anginal pain; whether it arises from the wall of the coronary artery or from some part of the heart itself still remains a mystery. In some cases, silent ischemia may show up during a routine EKG or stress test, but not always. It is most often discovered during 24-hour portable EKG or Holter monitoring, but if the attacks are infrequent, they may never be detected.

If silent ischemia is diagnosed, medication may be required to dilate the coronary arteries. The physician may also recommend angioplasty, a surgical procedure in which a balloon attached to a catheter is used to open up an obstruction, or even cardiac bypass surgery, in which a surgeon takes a blood vessel from another part of the body and constructs a detour around the blocked section of the coronary artery.

Chapter 7

CARDIAC ARRHYTHMIA

MY patient Polly called me with a problem. Every time she gets tense, she feels a fluttering in her chest, "just like there's a fish flopping around inside." Then the feeling stops abruptly. The more anxious Polly becomes, the worse the fluttering gets. Polly was worried that her symptoms were being caused by a serious heart problem, but actually they were being caused by a very normal albeit annoying irregularity in the heartbeat called an arrhythmia. Some arrhythmias, like Polly's, are mild and benign. Others can be deadly. In fact, arrhythmias may cause as many as 400,000 deaths a year in the United States. People with certain types of arrhythmia are prone to form blood clots that can lodge in the arteries supplying blood to the rest of the body, like the carotids, which supply blood to the brain. Therefore, arrhythmias are also a major cause of stroke. In order to understand why arrhythmias are so dangerous, you must first understand the anatomy of a heartbeat.

The normal human heart beats on average about 72 times a minute. It speeds up when we exert ourselves without our needing to tell it to do so—a reflex activity—and it slows down in the same way when we rest again. The heartbeat is regulated by an electrical impulse that begins in the sinus node, or pacemaker, situated in the right atrium. It travels throughout the heart in an orderly fashion, triggering the contraction that pumps blood out of the heart.

It is this regular cardiac rhythm that keeps the blood flowing properly. If the heart develops an irregular rhythm, it can interfere with the distribution of blood throughout the body. And as we know, if the body's vital organs do not get enough oxygen and nutrients, they will not be able to function. In cases of lethal arrhythmias, the heart may stop pumping altogether. Without prompt intervention, death is a certainty.

People who develop arrhythmias may experience a variety of symptoms: dizziness, fainting, or palpitations (a sense of something fluttering or beating irregularly in the front of the chest). However, some people may not feel anything at all.

maker loses its control over the other cells. If part of the heart becomes damaged due to a heart attack or episodes of oxygen loss, it could affect the ability of the heart to generate and conduct the electrical impulse properly. Many cells in the heart have the ability to beat on their own. When things are working well, the cells follow the lead of the pacemaker. If for any reason the pacemaker ceases to function, or if the electrical impulse between the pacemaker and other heart cells becomes blocked, some cells may begin to beat on their own. In some cases, the heart could develop a competing pacemaker—a group of cells take over for the pacemaker. The heart is no longer able to produce one, strong, unified contraction. As a result, the pumping ability of the heart is weakened.

Sometimes the normal rhythm of the heart breaks down so completely that many small islands of tissue begin to beat nearly simultaneously and the rhythmic beating of the chambers, whether atria or ventricles, becomes completely disrupted. This is called fibrillation. Atrial fibrillation occurs when the cells in the atria or upper chambers lose their synchrony or rhythm. (Since people with atrial fibrillation are more likely to develop blood clots that can flow downstream and block the carotid artery, this disorder accounts for 15 percent of all strokes.) If the cells in the ventricles or lower chambers begin to beat chaotically, the arrhythmia is called ventricular fibrillation. Once the ventricles begin to fibrillate, they are no longer able to contract. Blood will begin to collect in the heart, and, because the chambers can't contract, the blood cannot be pumped out again. Unless the normal heart rate is restored, death will occur within a few minutes.

There are more subtle forms of arrhythmia that are often difficult to diagnose. For example, I have treated several elderly patients for a condition called sick sinus syndrome—that is, the pacemaker has started to wear out and slow down. Patients with this problem have very low pulse rates, often dropping to below 40. Although the heart continues to operate, it pumps much less blood per minute than before. As a result, the blood flow to the brain is reduced, and the patients begin to show signs of personality change. Typically, they appear confused and slow-witted; they lose their sense of humor and may even have nightmares. Often, this condition is dismissed as senility by younger people—doctors and family members alike—who assume that the older person's brain is failing.

But contrary to popular belief, losing your ability to think is not a natural part of the aging process. Sometimes a physical ailment can be at the root of the problem. Fortunately, in this case, the problem can be successfully treated, perhaps with the insertion of an artificial pacemaker. In fact, after proper therapy, I have seen a complete turnaround in these supposedly "senile" patients. If you have an elderly relative who appears to be confused and slowing down, ask her doctor to check her for sick sinus syndrome. Don't assume that age is responsible.

CARDIOVERSION

If someone develops a lethal arrhythmia—for example, a heart attack patient in the CCU suddenly goes into ventricular fibrillation—immediate action is required. Typically, the patient will be cardioverted; that is, a defibrillator will be used to deliver an electric shock to the heart. If things work well, the jolt of electricity should shock and quiet all the cells of the heart, allowing the sinus node to resume control of the heart's rhythm. Once the pacemaker reestablishes its authority, the heart should begin beating normally.

ARTIFICIAL PACEMAKER

If the pacemaker is flawed to begin with, or the conduction pathway is interrupted, an artificial pacemaker may be needed to regulate the heartbeat. An artificial pacemaker is a small, battery-operated unit that produces electrical impulses. It is inserted in a pocket under the skin in the chest or upper abdomen. A pacemaker has two leads that are attached to the heart. Electrical impulses flow from these tiny wires to the heart, stimulating the heart and causing it to contract. In many cases, the artificial pacemaker will be able to take over for the real one, and the heart will once again work properly. The procedure is performed in the hospital and the patient may be able to go home the same day.

There are many different kinds of pacemakers and each must be individually tailored to the patient's needs. Some completely usurp the role of the sinus node, whereas others—called demand pacemakers—take charge only when the sinus node fails to function. When pacemakers first came into vogue in the early 1970s, patients were warned that the electronic wave transmissions by microwave ovens or electronic cash registers could interfere with their electrical charge. But today's pacemakers are no longer vulnerable to outside electrical fields.

If you have a pacemaker, make sure that you write down the model and year of insertion and carry it with you at all times. In fact, you might consider wearing a medic alert bracelet that notifies medical personnel you are wearing a pacemaker and gives other pertinent information. Although most pacemakers now have a life span of up to 15 years, like any other appliance, they can develop problems. Therefore, anyone with a pacemaker should monitor her pulse daily (ask your doctor what your normal range should be) and should also watch for signs of failure including unusual signs of bloating or swelling in ankles or legs, dizziness, fainting, heart palpitations, and difficulty breathing. If you have any of these symptoms, or suspect that your pacemaker may not be functioning properly, call your doctor.

ANTIARRHYTHMIC MEDICATION

Medication is often used to control irregularities of the heartbeat. Different classes of drugs work differently: Some slow the speed of conduction of the electrical impulse through the heart; others affect different parts of the conducting system in quite specific ways.

All antiarrhythmic drugs restore the electrical stability of the heart by slowing or extinguishing abnormal cardiac beats or rhythms. These drugs are divided into four different groups:

Class I: These drugs work by making the heart cell less excitable, that is, less likely to begin beating on its own. Class I drugs include Lidocaine, Quinidine, and flecainide (Tambocor). Administration of these drugs must be monitored very closely to make sure that they are not depressing the normal electrical activity of the heart as they correct or slow the abnormal rhythm. They may also cause gastrointestinal disturbances and should be used carefully in combination with drugs like digitalis.

Class II: These drugs, which include propanalol and atenolol, are beta blockers that run interference with hormones produced by the sympathetic nervous system. These drugs slow the heartbeat and can cause fatigue and low blood pressure.

Class III: These drugs, which include amiodarone (Cordarone) and bretylium, slow down the irritable heart cell's return to the resting state, in which it can be stimulated to beat. Thus, it is less likely to beat spontaneously again before a normal beat is generated. Side effects may include light sensitivity— patients on these drugs often see halos around lights at night—and thyroid problems. Class III drugs must be given carefully in patients who are taking blood thinners or digitalis.

Class IV: These drugs, which include verapamil and diltiazem, are calcium channel blockers. They also cause the heart to beat less forcefully and should be used with care in patients who are in heart failure.

Antiarrhythmic drugs are very powerful and must be precisely administered. It is not enough for the physician simply to hand the patient a prescription for a standard dose—treatment must be individually tailored to the patient. Unfortunately, some physicians don't take the time to prescribe these drugs correctly. A case in point is the mother of a friend of mine who had recently developed atrial fibrillation. Her physician prescribed Quinidine, an antiarrhythmic drug, in the usual dose. Within a few minutes after the first dose, the woman fainted; she had an unusual response to the drug that caused her blood pressure to drop.

Quinidine, or any antiarrhythmic medication, must be carefully introduced to the patient. If the patient can't tolerate the drug, or if the dose prescribed is too strong, the patient may experience serious side effects. If your doctor doesn't carefully monitor you in the initial phases of your taking these drugs, she may miss a problem until it is too late to do anything about it.

Despite the potential pitfalls, antiarrhythmic drugs can be very effective. For example, I have had good results with digitalis, a drug that strengthens the pumping action of the heart. But digitalis must be administered carefully and selectively—it is not for everyone. Any physician who uses digitalis must be aware that the drug is metabolized by the liver and excreted by the kidneys. If this drug is given to someone whose kidneys are not functioning properly, very high blood concentrations with ordinary doses of the drug may result, producing an accidental overdose.

As you can see, the pharmacology of the treatment of arrhythmias is extremely complex. Only skilled, experienced practitioners should use these drugs. And no matter who is prescribing the medication, close monitoring of the patient is essential. How can a patient determine if a physician is qualified? Your only recourse is to ask questions—lots of them. If your doctor wants you or a family member to take an antiarrhythmic medication, ask the following:

1. What is this drug for?
2. How much experience has the physician had with this particular medication?
3. Is a test dose required? If not, why?
4. What are the potential side effects?
5. How is the medication metabolized and eliminated by the body?
6. Why did you use this specific treatment?
7. Are there any foods, drugs, etc. that should not be used in combination with this drug?

If your doctor appears knowledgeable and has had good experience with this medication, chances are that she has given proper thought to her prescription.

If your questions are not answered to your satisfaction, seek a second opinion. Doing so is well within your rights as a patient.

SURGERY

If after an electrophysiologic study, the arrhythmia can be isolated to a portion of the heart, it may be possible to surgically remove or destroy that trouble-some part of the heart muscle to restore normal rhythm. If surgery is not indicated, doctors may use a procedure called catheter ablation to deliver an electrical shock to that area of the heart that is fibrillating. If neither of these treatments is possible, there's a new and innovative approach to this problem: the automatic implantable cardioverter defibrillator (AICD).

Similar to the pacemaker, this device is implanted under a pocket of skin, usually in the abdominal region. When the arrhythmia occurs, the portable defibrillator gives the heart a shock until normal rhythm is restored. In light of the difficulties in treating some arrhythmia with medication, although still experimental, the portable defibrillator offers a ray of hope.

RESOURCES: See also page 233.

Chapter 8

CONGENITAL HEART DEFECTS

ABOUT 500,000 American adults—more women than men—are born with some form of congenital heart disease, that is, defects in the anatomy of the heart that occur during its development. Although we don't know exactly why more women are born with heart defects, some obstetricians suspect that female fetuses are stronger than male fetuses and therefore more likely to survive abnormalities. Less than 10 percent of these abnormalities are genetic, and only 2 percent are caused by maternal exposure to either a virus, such as rubella, or a potentially toxic substance, such as alcohol. The rest are probably caused by a combination of factors, including a complex interaction between environment and genetics. About 1 out of 100 babies will be born with some kind of heart defect, and with proper treatment, most will go on to lead a relatively normal life. In rare cases involving extremely serious abnormalities, despite our best efforts, the infant may not survive beyond a few weeks.

Before the days of sophisticated diagnostic tests, infants with certain kinds of congenital defects would be born blue, gasping for breath, and no one would know specifically what was causing the problem or what to do about it. Needless to say, the prognosis was not good. Developed in the 1950s, cardiac catheterization enabled us actually to look inside the heart to see exactly which vessels or sections of the heart were defective. Although catheterization is a wonderful diagnostic tool, it is not without risk, especially for infants. Fortunately, today, we are able to diagnose most congenital problems in children with noninvasive procedures—those that don't require doctors to insert an instrument or catheter into a blood vessel or to operate on the patient. One such diagnostic tool is the Doppler echocardiogram, which uses sound waves to create an image of the heart's internal workings. X rays and blood tests are also used to help make a diagnosis.

There are many different types of heart defects—in fact, I could write a whole book on the subject. But here I will discuss only the most common defects and how they can be managed. By the way, *management* is the key word here: Anyone who has a child with a congenital heart defect, or who has one herself, should be carefully monitored by her physician. If a child is born with a heart defect, she should be carefully monitored by a pediatric cardiologist who specializes in these disorders. Many of the problems associated with heart defects that crop up later in life can be avoided, but the physician caring for the patient has to know when and how to intervene with therapy or corrective surgery.

In general, congenital heart defects fall into one of two categories: They either obstruct the flow of blood in the heart or blood vessels, or they cause the blood to flow through the heart abnormally. Depending on the anatomy of the defect, blood flow can be obstructed, rerouted to the wrong place, or can be ineffective because of incompetent valves. For example, if forward blood flow is impeded by a narrowing in a vessel, the flow of blood can be slowed down so much that it is unable to handle the body's needs. If a valve doesn't close properly, or there's a hole somewhere in the septa that divide the upper and the lower chambers of the heart from one another, blood may leak across the defect and flow in directions that are quite opposite to where it should be headed. This defect is called a shunt.

Depending on the degree of the problem, the defect could have severe consequences, or it could go unnoticed until an astute physician picks up an abnormal murmur, or until a patient begins to experience symptoms later in life. The following sections describe some of the more common heart defects.

MITRAL VALVE PROLAPSE

I recently had a thirty-five-year-old patient who believed that she was either going crazy or slowly dying from a mysterious, dreadful disease. Wendy had already been to four other doctors including two internists, a neurologist, and a psychiatrist. None of them could find anything physically wrong with her.

Within the past five years, Wendy's life had been made a nightmare by a series of terrifying episodes that followed a specific pattern: First, there would be a burning, tingling sensation in her neck. It would be followed by a feeling that she found hard to describe, but seemed to be a sense of being in a dream, or of unreality—a phenomenon known as depersonalization. These episodes often produced a feeling of panic of increasing intensity that culminated in the certainty that she was going to die. Although these episodes were infrequent, Wendy lived in dread of them, and as a result she had severely curtailed her activities. The once vivacious and ambitious investment banker had become so timid that she was afraid to drive her car or go to the supermarket for fear that she would have an episode in public.

Before I began the official examination, I chatted casually with Wendy about her family, her work, and her life before these episodes started occurring. I was struck by the fact that she seemed very intelligent and rational, and I began to wonder if the other doctors had overlooked a possible physical cause for her problem.

It didn't take a great deal of detective work to solve this mystery. Within a few minutes after I began the physical exam, I had a probable diagnosis. When I put my stethoscope on Wendy's chest to listen to her heart, there it was: the distinctive click and murmur typical of a common congenital condition known as mitral valve prolapse (MVP). To make sure that I was right, I then listened again as Wendy stood, squatted, stood up again, laid flat on her back first with her legs straight and then with her legs raised. An echocardiogram confirmed the diagnosis.

I was delighted to be able to tell Wendy that her problem wasn't in her head—it was in her heart. And it wasn't even that serious a problem. In fact, millions of other perfectly healthy people have it—including me.

MVP is an abnormality in the valve that guards the opening between the atrium, the left upper chamber of the heart, and the ventricle, the left lower chamber. The mitral valve consists of two flaps or leaflets that are anchored by guide wires to tiny, strong buttons or nubbins of muscle called papillary muscles. When the blood leaves the atrium, it flows through the mitral valve into the left ventricle. If everything is working properly, when the ventricle contracts the mitral valve should snap shut tightly and smoothly to prevent blood from seeping back into the atrium. In MVP, for some reason, the valve leaflets become enlarged and misshapen, billowing like sails full of wind back up into the left atrium when the ventricle contracts. Instead of closing smoothly, they allow blood to leak backward into the atrium. It is the regurgitation of blood back into the atrium that causes the distinctive murmur of this disorder.

MVP is the most common of all congenital heart defects, affecting twice as many women as men. At least 6 percent of all women—and about 17 percent of all women between the ages of twenty and forty—have MVP. Although we don't know what causes it, we do know that it tends to run in families and probably develops sometime during the fifth to eighth week of fetal development. Many people with MVP have no symptoms at all and may be completely unaware of it, although in most cases, it should be detected during a thorough physical exam.

About half of all prolapse patients complain of heart palpitations or skipped beats. Many experience mild chest pain, which is thought to be due to a stretching of the guide wires holding the mitral valve leaflets, resulting in decreased oxygen to the papillary muscles. Although this pain can sometimes be confused with angina, it is usually not as severe, nor can it be relieved by nitroglycerine. In some cases, patients may complain of occasional shortness of breath, light-headedness, dizziness, fainting, or numbness. These symptoms should be reported to a doctor immediately—especially if they're frequent or very severe—because they could be a result of small strokes that can occur due to an embolism from small blood clots or bacterial infection on the abnormal leaflets.

Finally, like my patient Wendy, a handful of prolapse patients complain of panic or anxiety attacks that are often mistaken for psychiatric problems. In some cases, antianxiety medication can alleviate the symptoms; however, in Wendy's case, drug therapy was unnecessary. Once Wendy understood the physical source of her problem, she was able to cope with it. The episodes that once terrified her no longer seemed to be so threatening, and Wendy was able to get on with her life.

Everyone can make a mistake and doctors are no exception. Even the best of doctors will tell you that medicine is not a perfect science. But I have a nagging suspicion that some may be just a little too willing to attribute a woman's complaints to female anxiety or hysteria, and therefore they neglect to look for other more probable causes.

While we're on the subject of female stereotypes, some doctors suggest that there is a typical profile of an MVP woman. According to these researchers, the typical prolapse woman is slim with low blood pressure, but she is also high-strung, nervous, and has above-average intelligence. I don't fully buy into this or any other stereotype—and I am especially wary when researchers, who are mostly male, conclude that a woman is the "nervous type"—but from a diagnostic standpoint, this information may be useful to alert a doctor to the possibility that someone may be "prolapse prone."

Most prolapse patients lead a perfectly normal life. However, there is one major complication of which MVP patients should be aware: They are at greater risk of developing bacterial endocarditis, a potentially dangerous infection of the mitral valve leaflets. Therefore, I advise my prolapse patients to take antibiotics before undergoing any "dirty" procedure that can introduce bacteria into the bloodstream. This consideration is especially important for dental work, any kind of examination of the gastrointestinal tract (like colonoscopy), and even childbirth.

There are some other serious albeit very rare complications associated with MVP. These include stroke or even the risk of sudden death due to a serious arrhythmia, or interruption in the normal beating action of the heart. However, these complications are very unusual. I caution all women, but especially those with MVP, not to use cocaine, because the drug has a tendency to produce serious disturbances in the rhythm of the heartbeat. It can be lethal, especially in women with MVP who may already be prone to arrhythmia. About 5 percent of all prolapse patients at some point in their lives require surgery to repair the valve.

Until the development of sophisticated diagnostic tools such as the echocardiogram, MVP remained a poorly understood disorder. Although we were able to detect the murmur with our stethoscopes, we were not able to pinpoint exactly what was causing it. After the initial discovery of MVP, early studies found that as much as 20 percent of the population had prolapses, but now that we have fine-tuned our diagnostic ability, we know that was a gross exaggeration. More sophisticated diagnostic procedures can help us distinguish between subtle variations of the norm and bona fide MVP.

We also know that some cases of prolapse are more serious than others. In fact, a recent ground-breaking study done by doctors at Massachusetts General Hospital examined 456 MVP patients. The study revealed that only 18 percent of these patients had both significant thickening of the mitral valve leaflets and leaflets that were so enlarged that they didn't close properly. The physicians concluded that the patients with both problems had "classic MVP" and were at greater risk of developing complications such as stroke than patients with just overgrown leaflets. If you were diagnosed with MVP before 1985, you should probably have another echocardiogram to assess the seriousness of your problem.

Although most people will never require treatment for MVP, some may need antiarrhythmic drugs if they are continually bothered by palpitations. Those with panic attacks may need medication to help prevent or control them. In my experience, however, I have found that once patients know exactly what is causing their feelings of fear and apprehension, they are often able to alleviate their symptoms on their own.

PATENT DUCTUS ARTERIOSUS

In the uterus, the fetus depends on the placental blood to deliver oxygen to its tissues, since it cannot breathe air in the liquid environment of the womb. In the fetus, therefore, the aorta and the pulmonary artery are connected by a channel called the ductus arteriosus. Most of the burden of pumping blood into the body of the fetus is done by the right ventricle rather than the left. But once out of the womb, the infant takes her first breath. Her lungs expand and must immediately take over the job of oxygenating the blood and removing its carbon dioxide and other waste products.

Within 24 to 48 hours after birth, the ductus arteriosus closes, but in rare cases—often involving premature birth—this doesn't happen. If the passageway remains open, some of the freshly oxygenated blood from the lungs that should go to the aorta to be fed to the rest of the body will instead flow back to the lungs. As a result of oxygen deprivation, the infant could tire easily, breathe rapidly, and be susceptible to lung infections or pneumonia. In some cases, infants with patent ductus arteriosus (PDA) may turn a slightly bluish color after birth, but in other cases, symptoms may not occur until several weeks later. Fortunately, once this defect is detected, it can be tied shut surgically without having to open the heart.

SEPTAL DEFECTS

The septum is the wall that separates the heart into the left and right sides. An atrial septal defect occurs if there is a hole in the septum separating the upper chambers of the heart. A ventricular septal defect refers to a hole in the tissue separating the lower chambers. If the defect between the two upper chambers or atria is large, a substantial amount of oxygenated blood from the lungs will flow across the defect into the right atrium rather than continuing on the normal route through the left ventricle out the aorta to deliver blood to the rest of the body.

Although with the aid of a stethoscope an observant pediatrician should be able to hear a heart murmur during a physical exam, this condition can go undetected for years because the child may have few if any symptoms. In some cases, a woman may not be aware of this problem until her thirties, when the murmur is first heard. It is quite common for someone to live well into her fifties or sixties without any symptoms. Suddenly, however, the patient becomes aware of increasing shortness of breath and an irregular cardiac rhythm. Once diagnosed, her physician will probably recommend surgical correction.

There are different kinds of atrial septal defects, and one of the most serious is the ostium primum, which also affects the structure of the mitral valve. By age thirty or forty, many of these patients develop atrial enlargement and arrhythmias. The condition then requires medication, and if possible, surgical repair.

VENTRICULAR SEPTAL DEFECTS

Normally, blood should flow from the left ventricle to the aorta and out to the rest of the body. But if there is a hole in the interventricular septum, the blood from the left side of the heart may flow into the right side and flow once again through the lungs. As a result, high blood pressure may develop in the vessels of the lungs, which may become permanent and cause lasting damage. Although some of the openings may close spontaneously after birth, open heart surgery may be needed to close the opening during childhood. Women with small ventricular septal defects can usually tolerate pregnancy well, but should be carefully watched for signs of increased shunting across the defect, or for signs of infection in the heart.

AORTIC STENOSIS

When blood from the left ventricle flows through the aortic valve into the aorta, the valve should snap close to prevent the flow of blood from seeping backward in the ventricle. A normal aortic valve consists of three filmy pieces of connective tissue or leaflets. In some cases, however, the valve has an abnormal number of leaflets—usually two, but sometimes as many as four or as few as one. In these cases, the valve leaflets thicken and even calcify and fuse, eventually narrowing and blocking the flow of blood out of the ventricle. No one knows why this happens.

Usually, there are no symptoms until middle age. Typically, the patient will begin to have angina, arrhythmias, or periods of unconsciousness. She may first go into congestive heart failure and experience shortness of breath and cough, and eventually go into pulmonary edema (fluid in the lungs). Fortunately, aortic stenosis can be successfully treated by opening up the stiff leaflets surgically. Sometimes an artificial valve may be needed if the original valve cannot be repaired.

In other cases, a new procedure called balloon valvuloplasty may be used to open the valve. A special catheter containing a balloon is placed across the constricted or narrowed valve and then inflated to stretch open the valve. This same treatment can be used for other stenosed valves of the heart and is a wonderful addition to what we can do for patients with this kind of problem.

PULMONARY STENOSIS

The blood flows from the right ventricle through the pulmonary valve to the lungs. If the pulmonary valve is too narrow, the right ventricle will pump harder to push the blood through. The hardworking ventricle thickens and contracts more slowly in order to compensate for the heavy load it must bear. If the valve is very tight, blood flow to the oxygen-giving lung is so poor that the patient may appear bluish in color, a sign of oxygen deprivation. If the pressure against which the ventricle must pump is too high, the valve may be opened surgically or by balloon valvuloplasty.

TETRALOGY OF FALLOT

This disorder consists of several anatomic defects in the heart: a large hole in the septum that divides ventricles; a narrowing of the pulmonic valve; and an aorta that "overrides" both ventricles, allowing blood from both the left and the right circulations to be pumped forward into the aorta. As a result, blood flows from the right to the left side of the heart, both across the hole in the septum and into the aorta. Thus, "blue" unoxygenated blood is fed to the body and the child has a bluish discoloration of the skin that is particularly pronounced in the lips, tongue, and tips of the fingers and toes. Surgery is often required to allow the child to grow properly and have a normal life span.

COARCTATION OF THE AORTA

The aorta is the main artery that carries blood from the heart to the body. In cases of coarctation of the aorta, this vital artery is pinched or constricted, blocking the flow of blood from the heart to the lower part of the body. In rare cases, this condition can cause high blood pressure. If the coarctation is beyond the place where the artery supplying the right side of the head and arm originates, the blood pressure in the right arm can be very high, while that in the left arm is normal. Similarly, if the constriction is still further along, pressures in the arms can be high, while that in the legs can be normal. Any patient being assessed for high blood pressure should have the pressures recorded in both arms and in the legs. If the coarctation is severe enough, the left ventricle is eventually overwhelmed and the patient goes into congestive heart failure. In some cases, the aorta may need to be surgically repaired; in rare cases, balloon angioplasty can be used to relieve the constriction.

Having a child born with a congenital heart defect—or discovering that you have one yourself—can be very frightening. But keep in mind that there are more than half a million Americans living today with various types of heart defects and with proper medical attention the prognosis is extremely good for most of them.

As I said earlier, anyone with a heart defect should be carefully monitored by her doctor. In addition, patients with certain defects, especially those affecting valves, should be aware that they are more prone to endocarditis, or bacterial infection of the heart. Therefore, to avoid any problems, they should take antibiotics before dental work, any kind of surgical or invasive diagnostic procedure, during and immediately after childbirth.

With improved noninvasive diagnostic procedures such as Dopplers and new nonsurgical procedures such as balloon valvuloplasty, the outlook for the diagnosis and treatment of congenital heart disease is getting brighter all the time.

IV

THE WOMAN AT RISK
FOR HEART ATTACK

Chapter 9

PROFILE OF THE
HIGH-RISK WOMAN

My father had a heart attack at fifty. His cholesterol has always been extremely high. My mother's sister died of a sudden heart attack at thirty-nine. My cholesterol has always been on the high end. Believe me, I'm worried. I watch what I eat—I stick to fish, vegetables, never anything fried or fatty. I exercise all the time. In fact, I bought a Nordic Track for my home so I can work out every day. I know that I'm at high risk for heart disease, but I'm doing everything that I can to make sure that it doesn't happen to me.

—Lynn, thirty-eight years old

A risk factor is any activity or trait that increases your chances of developing a specific disease—in this case, coronary artery disease, or CAD. In Lynn's case, family history of heart disease and high cholesterol increase her risk of developing CAD. Chances are that many of you reading this book will also have one or more risk factors for developing CAD. Perhaps, like Lynn, one of your parents or close relatives died at an early age from a heart attack. Family history of heart disease—your heredity—is a leading risk factor for CAD because there is a chance that you may have inherited the characteristic or trait that contributed to your relative's heart attack. Or, perhaps your lifestyle puts you at greater jeopardy for heart disease.

Before you panic, let me remind you of an important fact. Just because you may fall into the high-risk category it doesn't automatically mean that your fate is sealed: that somewhere, sometime, you are going to have a heart attack. For one thing, despite the spectacular technological advances in medicine over the past decades, there's still a lot we don't know. One of the things we can't predict with 100 percent accuracy is who will develop heart disease and who will enjoy a lifetime of good health. All we do know is that women who share certain characteristics are more likely to develop heart disease than others. In addition, we now know that even women with a number of strikes against them can beat the odds by making positive changes in their lifestyle.

PHYSICAL CHARACTERISTICS

Age

As a rule, the older you are, the greater your risk of CAD. Until age thirty, accidents are the leading cause of death in women. From age thirty to forty, cancer becomes the number one killer of women, with accidental death running second. From age forty to sixty, cancer still leads, but heart disease is now in second place. By age sixty, men and women are at equal risk for heart disease, and by age sixty-five, heart disease becomes the leading cause of death in women.

Menopausal State

In women, age is not the only issue. Regardless of her age, once menstruation ceases, a woman's risk of developing CAD increases between twofold and threefold. In fact, women who have had premenopausal hysterectomies also have a threefold risk increase of CAD.

Body Build: Comparing Pears and Apples

Women who are officially defined as obese—that is, who are between 20 percent and 30 percent over their ideal body weight—are at greater risk of developing CAD. In fact, according to a recent eight-year study done at Harvard Medical School and the Brigham and Women's Hospital, a significant amount of heart disease among women is attributable to being overweight. This study followed 115,886 U.S. women who were age thirty to fifty-five in 1976 and free of any signs of heart disease. Out of this group, 605 developed some form of CAD. According to the study, as much as 70 percent of the CAD among obese women, and 40 percent of CAD among women overall, is related to excess weight.

However, several other studies have noted that overall obesity is not as important a risk factor as is the distribution of the excess fat on the body. People who are round in the middle or shaped like apples are at greater risk than people who are shaped like pears, where the weight is concentrated on their bottom half. Studies show that midsection obesity—the so-called spare tire—which is more common in men, is far more dangerous than fat concentrated on the hips and thighs, which is more typical of women. Recent studies also suggest that women with the thickest skin folds due to obesity have the lowest rates of HDL—the good cholesterol—and therefore run a greater risk of heart disease. In addition, overweight women run a greater risk of diabetes and high blood pressure, which also increases their risk of heart attack. Women who keep their weight within normal limits have the lowest rate of heart disease.

Another recent study suggests that shortness may be at the very least a minor risk factor for CAD. According to researchers at Boston University School of Public Health, women who are 4′ 11″ or under are at a 50 percent greater risk of heart attack than women who are at least 5′ 4″. However, since shorter women are more likely to carry their weight at midsection than taller ones, height may be less important than overall body shape.

MEDICAL HISTORY

Family History of Coronary Artery Disease

If you have a father who has had a heart attack before the age of fifty-six, or a mother who has had one before the age of sixty, you have an increased risk of developing CAD. The younger the age of your parent or grandparent's first heart attack, the greater your risk.

Elevated Blood Lipids

HIGH TRIGLYCERIDES.

Triglycerides are a type of fat that can be found in the blood serum and measured by a special test. According to the Framingham study, women with higher than normal levels of triyglycerides—a three-time fasting level of more than 190 mg/dl—were at significantly greater risk of developing CAD than others. Interestingly enough, high triglycerides do not appear to be a risk factor for men until levels approach 400 mg/dl.

HIGH CHOLESTEROL.

Cholesterol is a waxy, fatlike substance found in the blood serum. Women typically have higher cholesterol levels than men. However, studies are not consistent in pinpointing the exact level of blood cholesterol that is dangerous for women. For example, Framingham showed that in women with cholesterol levels of 265 mg/dl or higher there was a significant increase in heart disease. Another study by the Lipid Research Clinics reported that women with cholesterol levels higher than 235 mg/dl had a 70 percent greater risk of death than women with lower levels. I believe that depending on other risk factors even a cholesterol of 235 mg/dl may be too high. However, barring other risk factors, under proper circumstances a cholesterol of up to 240 mg/dl may be acceptable for a woman.

A lot depends on which type of cholesterol is the predominant cholesterol: high-density lipoproteins (HDL) or low-density lipoproteins (LDL). HDL is often referred to as the "good" cholesterol because it may help prevent arteriosclerosis. LDL, known as the "bad" cholesterol, may actually promote clogging of the arteries. Many researchers believe that the overall cholesterol level is not nearly as good a predictor of heart disease in women as the level of HDL versus LDL. Ideally, your HDL-to-LDL ratio should be no more than 4:1. For example, if your HDL is 40 and your LDL is 120, the ratio is 3:1, which is excellent. However, if your HDL is 30 and your LDL is 180, the ratio is 6:1, which is considered poor. Fortunately, women typically have higher levels of HDL than men and better HDL-to-LDL ratios.

The rule of thumb for everyone is that HDL cholesterol should be higher than 35 mg/dl and LDL cholesterol should be lower than 130 mg/dl. The average woman has an HDL cholesterol level of 40 mg/dl.

In women, HDL drops after menopause, and LDL rises, which undoubtedly contributes to the increased rate of CAD. Women with elevated LDL are at greater risk of developing heart disease.

Diabetes

We learned from the Framingham study that women with diabetes—the inability to metabolize properly sugar or glucose—are at double risk of having a heart attack than nondiabetic women. In fact, diabetic women of any age run the same risk as their male counterparts of having a myocardial infarction.

For some reason, diabetic women do not enjoy the same protection that other premenopausal women have against heart disease. Many diabetic women have higher blood pressure and blood cholesterol levels than nondiabetic women. They also have other circulatory problems that can contribute to the onset of CAD. Depending on the type of diabetes, the condition can be controlled through diet, medication, or both. With proper treatment the prognosis for diabetics is greatly improved.

High Blood Pressure

Blood pressure is the force exerted by the blood against the arterial walls. Between 50 and 60 million Americans—nearly half of them women—have high blood pressure, that is, blood pressure above the average 120/80. The top number represents the systolic pressure, the pressure when the heart contracts and pushes blood through the arteries. The bottom number represents the diastolic pressure, the pressure in the arteries when the heart muscle relaxes between beats.

Women with elevated blood pressure run a greater risk of developing stroke, kidney disease, and heart disease. As a woman ages, her chances of developing high blood pressure become greater than a man's. If you have a parent or grandparent with high blood pressure, or if you became hypertensive during pregnancy, you are also at risk of developing hypertension later in life. High blood pressure is such an important risk factor that I have devoted chapter 10 to this topic, which I advise all women to read.

Proteinuria, or Protein in the Urine

During your annual physical, your doctor should take a fresh urine specimen in which she checks for, among other things, the presence of protein. Proteinuria indicates that the kidneys are not functioning properly, due to damage caused by one of a number of diseases, including hypertension. Whatever the cause, proteinuria is a red flag that should not be ignored.

Enlarged Heart

When the left ventricle of the heart is overworked due to high blood pressure, obesity, or other problems, the heart wall thickens. In part, this is due to the fact that the hardworking muscle cells become enlarged to accommodate the extra workload. The condition is called left ventricular hypertrophy. Left ventricular hypertrophy can be diagnosed by an echocardiogram, a simple noninvasive test in which sound waves are sent to and reflected from the heart and other tissues. The resulting pattern produces a very detailed picture of the anatomy of the heart and valves. Studies show that an enlarged heart greatly increases a woman's risk of heart attack and should be taken very seriously.

Increased Fibrinogen Levels

Fibrinogen is a substance produced in the body that is necessary for the proper clotting of blood when injury occurs. Fibrinogen levels are typically higher in women than in men, but increased levels of fibrinogen have been associated with higher than normal rates of CAD. Smokers tend to have higher levels of fibrinogen than nonsmokers.

High Hematocrit Level

Hematocrit, the percentage of the total blood volume made up of red blood cells, can be measured by a simple blood test. A higher than normal level has been associated with sudden death syndrome—death without prior evidence of CAD. A high hematocrit could mean that the tissues of the body are being deprived of oxygen, an early sign of arteriosclerosis or narrowing of the arteries.

Five or More Pregnancies

A new study reports that women who have had five or more children have lower levels of HDL, which puts them at greater risk of falling victim to CAD. Although we can't say for certain that many pregnancies are a serious risk factor, it's probably a good idea for women with many children to pay particular attention to their blood lipid levels.

LIFESTYLE

Smoking

Twenty-seven percent of all women smoke. Although the overall rate of smoking is on the decline, women are not quitting as rapidly as men. For example, from 1965 to 1987, smoking declined among men by nearly 20 percent. During the same period, only 6 percent of all women smokers stopped. In fact, one recent study showed that more high school senior girls are smoking than senior boys. Smoking wreaks havoc on a woman's body, as illustrated by the fact that more women today die of lung cancer than breast cancer. Smokers also run an increased risk of heart attack and stroke. Oddly enough, smokers develop a distinctive type of arteriosclerotic lesion that is not found in nonsmokers.

In addition, smokers become menopausal two to three years earlier than nonsmokers, which also increases their risk of developing heart disease. Young women who smoke have lower levels of the beneficial HDL and higher levels of the harmful LDL than nonsmokers, and women who smoke are more likely to develop severe malignant hypertension than those who don't.

Substance Abuse

There are approximately 4,595,000 women who are alcoholics or are alcohol dependent in the United States. Substance abuse experts also note a dramatic surge in the usage of cocaine and crack among women. Both substances are highly toxic to the heart, especially for women. Cocaine use during pregnancy is especially dangerous for the infant. Women who take cocaine during pregnancy are 10 to 15 times more likely to give birth to a baby with a serious heart defect. According to one recent study, as many as 10 percent of all pregnant women may use cocaine. For more information on dangerous addictions and heart disease, read chapter 13.

Birth Control Pills

Studies show that women who use oral contraceptives are more likely to develop hypertension and stroke than those who don't. In fact, 5 percent of all women on the pill develop a blood pressure of 140/90 or greater. Only 50 percent of these elevated pressures return to normal after going off the pill. Women who smoke and take the pill run a 30 percent to 40 percent increase of developing CAD. To smoke *and* take the pill is playing with dynamite.

Lack of Physical Activity

Women who lead a sedentary life with little or no physical activity are at three times the risk of developing heart disease as those who don't. Women who engage in even the most moderate type of exercise—those who walk a half hour a day at least three days a week—have a lower resting heart rate, which could protect them against heart attack. Exercise provides a great release for stress. (For more information, read chapter 18.)

The Role of Stress

Unrelenting stress can have a toxic effect on the body for both men and women, and I believe it is a leading contributor to the development of CAD. However, most of the research done on stress and heart disease has focused on men, specifically on the type A personality—the aggressive, competitive go-getter who takes the fast track all the way to the cardiac care unit. Books have been written about him, and medical journals and popular magazines have devoted countless pages to discussing his plight. Although there has been considerably less attention focused on women and stress, Framingham and a handful of recent studies suggest that many women—especially those with multiple roles at work and at home—are under extreme stress, the kind that raises blood pressure and increases their risk of developing CAD. Based on my personal experiences with patients, I have identified six types of women who I believe are at the greatest risk of ending up as cardiac patients. To find out if you are one of them, read chapter 12.

*   *   *

If you have one or more risk factors for CAD, talk to your doctor about ways of minimizing your risk. When it comes to heart disease, I firmly believe in the adage, "Forewarned is forearmed." If you know that there is something in your medical history or lifestyle that increases the odds of your getting a heart attack or a stroke, it is critical that you do everything in your power to prevent this from happening. With your doctor's help, it may be possible to substantially tip the odds in your favor.

Chapter 10

HIGH BLOOD PRESSURE:
THE SILENT KILLER

HIGH blood pressure, or hypertension, is one of the most common risk factors for CAD; it is also one of the most misunderstood. High blood pressure is often called the "silent killer" for good reason. It does its dirty work quietly—so quietly in fact that the victim is usually totally unaware of what is happening to her body. Because you usually don't feel sick, it's easy to ignore high blood pressure and pretend that it isn't there. But whether you acknowledge it or not, the damage is being done. A decade or two down the road, there may be a very steep price to pay for your neglect. If untreated, this invisible, symptomless disease can cause kidney failure, eye damage, heart attack, and stroke.

Before I discuss how to diagnose and treat high blood pressure, let me first define it. Blood pressure measures the force exerted by the blood against the arterial wall. Blood pressure values depend on age, sex, and other factors. Older people tend to have higher pressures due to a stiffening or hardening of their arteries.

However, even among younger women there is a tremendous variability in blood pressure. A normal premenopausal woman usually has a blood pressure of anywhere between 110/65 and 120/80. The top number measures the systolic pressure, which is generated when the heart contracts and pushes blood into the artery. The bottom number is the diastolic pressure, or the pressure in the arteries when the heart muscle relaxes between beats.

According to a 1988 report issued by the National Institutes of Health, if the diastolic pressure is less than 90, a systolic pressure of 140 or less is considered normal. However, a systolic reading of 140 to 159 would be considered "borderline isolated systolic hypertension," and anything higher than 160 is "isolated systolic hypertension." The same report said that a diastolic pressure of less than 85 is normal. Diastolic pressures of 85 to 89 are considered the high end of normal, 90 to 104 is mild hypertension, 105 to 114 is moderate hypertension, and 115 and higher is considered to be severe hypertension.

For an adult woman, anything less than 140/90 is considered within normal range. In some cases, however, even a so-called normal pressure may be abnormal. For example, if a patient who has always had a pressure of 110/65 suddenly has a reading of 130/80, I would try to discover what, if anything, caused the increase. It could be that she is under a great deal of stress, or that she has eaten a particularly salty meal the night before her physical, which could temporarily raise her blood pressure. If, for example, the woman had just started oral contraceptives, I would be sure to monitor this patient very carefully for any further increases.

Depending on other risk factors, even the high end of normal may be too high for some people. In fact, a recent study done by researchers at the University of Michigan suggests that even slightly elevated blood pressures can be dangerous for some people, especially those who are obese—that is 20 percent to 30 percent above their recommended body weight. Borderline hypertension is defined as anywhere between 140 and 160 systolic, and between 90 and 95 diastolic. Anything above those levels is bona fide hypertension. (In elderly patients, however, systolic pressures are sometimes allowed to rise to 180 to compensate for aging arteries, as long as the patient doesn't have other risk factors such as obesity or high cholesterol.)

Blood pressures below the norm are not considered to be a problem as long as the organs are getting enough blood and the kidneys are able to function. However, extremely low pressures—those in which the systolic pressure drops below 80—will usually result in symptoms such as dizziness or fainting. Extremely low pressures are often a result of trauma to the body and the cause must be identified and treated immediately. For example, excessive blood loss or severe dehydration will cause the blood pressure to plummet as low as 60/40. Once the blood or fluid is replaced, the pressure should begin to return to normal.

As recently as the 1940s, a doctor could offer very little in terms of treatment to a patient with high blood pressure. Then came a major breakthrough: the introduction of a group of drugs called diuretics that were effective in lowering blood pressure in most people. In the 1970s and 1980s, research yielded a whole range of medications that work in different ways. Nowadays, in nearly all cases, high blood pressure can be treated safely and effectively with either medication, changes in lifestyle, or a combination of the two. When it comes to high blood pressure, as you will see, ignorance is the real enemy.

High blood pressure, or hypertension, is one of the most common ailments of the twentieth century. About 60 million Americans—one-fifth of the population—have elevated blood pressure. Perhaps as many as 50 percent of all African-Americans have hypertension. About 20 million Americans take medication for high blood pressure, making these drugs the most commonly prescribed medicines in the United States.

Until age fifty-five, women usually have lower blood pressures than men of the same age. After that, the tables suddenly turn. Between fifty-five and sixty-five women run the same risk as men of developing high blood pressure, but by age sixty-five they are even more likely than men to become hypertensive. Although hypertension appears to be a late-onset disease, it can also occur in children and even in infants.

In adults, about 95 percent of all cases of high blood pressure are called *essential* or *primary* hypertension, meaning that the cause is unknown. Diet, stress, and genetics—or a combination of the three—are factors that are believed to play a role in high blood pressure. But in most cases, we can't pinpoint the exact cause. The remaining 5 percent of cases are called *secondary* hypertension, meaning that the cause can be determined and often corrected so that the hypertension can be reversed.

THE CONSEQUENCES OF HIGH BLOOD PRESSURE

Although we don't know what causes most cases of high blood pressure, we do know the havoc it can wreak on the human body. As we discussed earlier, the heart pumps blood to all parts of the body through a vast network of blood vessels. The largest of these vessels are called arteries. Arteries merge with smaller vessels called arterioles, which in turn are connected with the capillaries. In cases of high blood pressure, the trouble begins in the arterioles, which have muscle cells within their walls. If these contract too much, the total volume of the system into which the heart ejects its blood is reduced and the pressure rises. The heart must work harder against the higher pressure. Over time, it can become enlarged—a sign of overwork—and will eventually fail under the strain. Any sudden exertion—an emotional shock or a physical challenge, such as running up a flight of steps—may be the proverbial straw that breaks the camel's back.

The heart is not the only organ that can be affected by hypertension. The kidneys suffer damage from high blood pressure and may eventually fail in their job of eliminating waste products from the blood efficiently. The arterioles themselves may become scarred and permanently narrowed by the increased pressure, making it harder to correct the condition. High blood pressure also damages the eyes; it can cause retinal hemorrhaging and even blindness. If the pressure in the arteries feeding the brain becomes too high, the blood vessel will give way and tear, resulting in a hemorrhagic stroke. People with high blood pressure are twice as likely to get heart attacks and eight times as likely to get strokes as the normal population, especially if they are over fifty-five.

A stroke can occur when the brain does not receive enough blood, and as a result portions of brain tissue die. Depending on the severity and location of the stroke, the victim may be left with severe neurological problems. These can affect speech, cause physical weakness or paralysis, and even impair the patient's ability to think. However, in many cases, often with the help of rehabilitative therapy, stroke victims can achieve a partial or even full recovery.

Because of their increased risk of stroke, I believe that patients with high blood pressure should be educated about the early warning signs of stroke, which include:

1. Dizziness or feelings of unsteadiness
2. Loss of speech or difficulty in talking or understanding speech
3. Loss of vision, especially in one eye
4. Any unexplained weakness or numbness in the face, arm, or leg on one side of the body

If you have any of these symptoms, notify your doctor at once or go to the nearest emergency room.

In some cases, people may experience some or all of these symptoms very briefly and then resume normal activity. This experience is called a transient ischemic attack (TIA). TIAs are important because very often they are early warning signs of a stroke. In fact, 50 percent of all patients with TIAs have a full-blown stroke within one year after the episode. In many cases, however, a stroke can be averted by prompt medical attention.

I'm not writing this to frighten the 60 million people with high blood pressure. In most cases, it takes a long time for hypertension to do its damage, and with proper treatment, none of these bad things have to happen in the first place.

In order to avoid running into any of these difficulties, you must first make sure that you aren't walking around with an undiagnosed case of high blood pressure. I hope by now I have convinced everyone who is reading this book of the importance of a thorough annual physical examination by a careful physician. There is simply no substitute for good preventive care. If you have been examined by your doctor on a regular basis, then you should already know whether your blood pressure is normal or not, and if it is high, you should be receiving appropriate treatment.

DIAGNOSIS

There may be other people, ranging from your Aunt Martha to the nice volunteer at the shopping mall, who may offer to take your blood pressure. And although these people may do the job very well, I feel that only your physician can make a true diagnosis of hypertension, or can totally eliminate the possibility of your having the disease. As you will see, there's a lot more to taking blood pressure than merely reading the numbers.

Blood pressure is measured with an instrument called a sphygmomanometer, or pressure gauge. The test itself is painless (although not as quick as most people believe) and noninvasive. Blood pressure should be taken by a doctor or a nurse in a quiet setting. A strip of fabric containing a rubber bladder (an empty rubber sac) is wrapped around the upper arm so that the bladder is over one of the large arteries in the area. The doctor then pumps air into the bladder until she can no longer hear the sound of the heart beating under the stethoscope. The sounds have stopped because the pressure from the bladder exceeds that in the artery, and no more blood flows in the vessel.

Then, as the doctor slowly allows the air to escape from the cuff, the pressure in the bladder decreases. At the point where the bladder pressure equals that in the artery, the blood once more begins to flow and the doctor can hear the sound of the blood pulsing through the artery. The pressure at which those sounds begin is called the systolic pressure. As the bladder continues to deflate, the sounds fade and finally cannot be heard any longer; the pressure at which this happens is called the diastolic pressure. The two readings are recorded on your chart. As we have explained, the systolic pressure measures the pressure in the artery at the moment the heart contracts and ejects the blood into the arteries. The diastolic pressure, the second number, measures the pressure in the vessels when the heart muscle is relaxed; it is the way the doctor measures the tone of the vessels.

A good reading depends on having a cuff of proper width and length. The standard cuff fits most adults, but a wider cuff is available for people with large arms. There is a special cuff for children.

Blood pressure is not static: It rises and falls throughout the day, almost second to second, depending on many factors. Therefore, it's critical that blood pressure be measured in a quiet, restful atmosphere. The doctor should take the pressure in both arms, and when the patient is lying down, sitting up, and standing erect. Sometimes it is important to measure blood pressure in the legs as well, particularly if the doctor suspects some blockage of flow in the arterial system to the lower part of the body. According to protocols issued by the American Heart Association, before a positive diagnosis of high blood pressure can be made the physician should repeat the test on three separate office visits. Each time she should get a reading of at least 150/90. Only then can she conclusively say, "You have high blood pressure."

What if only one or two of the readings were very high, or a patient only seems to get high blood pressure when she's in the doctor's office and nowhere else? For instance, I recently had a patient with a classic case of "white coat hypertension." Her blood pressure soared to 175/110 for the first reading, and

30 minutes later it was down to a safer 130/85. During the course of her examination, she confessed that she was terrified of doctors and was sure that her fear was causing her blood pressure to rise. She may have been right.

Although the relationship between stress and hypertension is not fully understood, when someone is frightened certain chemicals are released by the body that cause arteries that regulate the size of the vessels, called arterioles, to constrict, thus causing the surge in blood pressure. That is why some doctors dismiss a first-time reading as irrelevant, especially if they know that a patient is anxious in their office. But I feel that they are making a grave mistake. The patient who is frightened enough in her doctor's office to send her blood pressure soaring is going to get scared in other situations. Life is full of stressful surprises, and it doesn't make me feel any better to know that a patient only gets high blood pressure when she's nervous. If her blood pressure rises to the stratosphere when I put a cuff around her arm, you can bet that it's going to happen again when she's under a different kind of stress. I'm not saying that all cases of "white coat hypertension" require medication, but I certainly feel that people with this problem should at the very least be offered some help in terms of stress management.

About 80 percent of people with high blood pressure fall somewhere in the mild or borderline category. Not all of these people will be put on medication. If there are no other significant risk factors, a doctor may simply recommend that a patient get more exercise, lose weight if she needs to, cut down on salt (which may contribute to hypertension), and increase her intake of foods high in fiber such as fruits and grains. If the doctor feels that the patient is under a great deal of stress, she may recommend short-term therapy, especially if the hypertension first appears after a traumatic experience, such as a sudden death in the family or a divorce. Other patients may require antihypertensive medication.

After the diagnosis of high blood pressure is made, it is simply not enough to write a prescription and send the patient on her way. It is absolutely critical that the physician do a thorough follow-up examination to see if the elevated blood pressure has caused any damage to the most vulnerable organs: the heart, the kidneys, and the eyes. If any of these organs have been affected, special treatment will be required to prevent further damage. Although we can rarely find the cause of high blood pressure in adult patients, children are a different story: When a child's blood pressure is too high, we should always look for an underlying cause before dismissing it as essential or primary hypertension. In these cases, high blood pressure can be a symptom of another problem, such as a kidney disorder, which in most cases can be treated. Since high blood pressure is still fairly rare in adults under thirty-five, it is also well worth the effort to look a little harder in these cases. A detailed series of tests is indicated in any patient under thirty-five who has newly discovered high blood pressure and no family history of the disease.

Once I know for sure that a patient is hypertensive, I try to rule out as many causes as possible. First, if I get an elevated pressure after three readings in either arm, I take the blood pressure in the legs as well to check for a condition called coarctation of the aorta. The aorta is the great artery that carries the blood from the heart to the vessels supplying the rest of the body. If the aorta is narrowed somewhere along its course, the blood pressure may be increased in only one arm, and not at all in the legs.

I also listen to the neck with a stethoscope at various points in the body, particularly in the abdomen, to see if there are sounds of turbulent flow at the point where the large vessels branch off from the aorta to supply the kidneys. In the course of the examination, I use my ophthalmoscope to look into the patient's eyes at the vessels within. The back of the eye, or the retina, is a wonderful window through which to see whether or not those all-important arterioles are narrowed or structurally distorted. I also look for hemorrhages on the retina, which is another consequence of high blood pressure. I often refer patients with suspected damage to one of my colleagues, an ophthalmologist, so that he can make baseline observations with me. Together we assess the extent—and implications—of the problem and work out a treatment plan for the patient before her vision is harmed further.

I devote much of my time with the patient to listening to what she says and how she sounds. I take a complete family history. In the process, I try to find out as much about my patient as possible. Did her mother or father have hypertension? Do any of her siblings? Is she on any medication that could be raising her blood pressure, such as certain antihistamines, diet pills, or oral contraceptives? Is she on any antidepressants, which, in combination with the chemical tyramine that is found in some foods, could be raising her blood pressure? Does she eat a lot of licorice (another food known to cause hypertension and low serum potassium, particularly in African-Americans)? Does she have any symptoms, or a history of previous illnesses or a family history that might suggest a kidney problem or a hormonal imbalance? Is she under a great deal of stress?

After the physical is done, I do a urinalysis in my office on a specimen of urine the patient has just produced, to look for any red blood cells, which are often an early warning sign of kidney damage. By the time the urine is sent to a laboratory for further testing, these cells will have burst and there will be no evidence of this important symptom. I also take blood samples to send to a laboratory specifically to check the thyroid function: An overactive thyroid could cause high blood pressure. In addition, I order a complete blood lipid profile to determine cholesterol level: HDL/LDL ratios and triglycerides.

I then perform an EKG to see if there are any abnormalities in the anatomy of the heart or in the cardiac rhythm. Signs of ischemic heart disease, or oxygen deprivation—a sure indication of coronary arteriosclerosis—can also be picked up on this important test. If the EKG reveals any damage to the heart, I order an echocardiogram, which would confirm whether or not the ventricle has become enlarged as a result of the high blood pressure. Although an enlarged or thickened left ventricular chamber increases the patient's risk of developing heart disease and stroke, there are some new antihypertensive medications that may help reverse some of the damage. Needless to say, the medications will do no good unless you identify the patients who need them.

I admit that nine times out of ten, when dealing with adults, an exhaustive search for the cause of high blood pressure turns up nothing. When this is the case, I simply accept it and go on to devise a treatment plan. But in rare cases, particularly in patients under thirty-five who do not have a family history of hypertension, further testing, close observation, and even hospitalization may be warranted. In such cases it could be a constriction of the blood supply to one kidney or an overactive adrenal gland that is causing the problem. There might even be a malfunction of the pituitary gland. In most cases, these conditions can be corrected, either with surgery, medication, or both, and the high blood pressure returns to normal.

TREATMENT

Let's start with the easy part. If your diastolic pressure is consistently more than 105, there's no question about it: You should be taking medication to lower your blood pressure. But only 20 percent of all cases are this clear-cut. Most people with hypertension have a diastolic blood pressure between 90 and 104, and whether or not to prescribe drugs or to try other nonmedical alternatives is very much a judgment call on the part of the physician.

Sometimes medication is not the answer. A case in point is my patient Susan, a thirty-nine-year-old businesswoman who had slightly elevated blood pressure. After Susan took off a few pounds and joined a health club, her blood pressure dropped to a normal level. However, it began creeping upward again after she got married. The relationship was fine, but the living arrangements left a lot to be desired. Unwilling to give up her lucrative job, Susan lived in New Jersey and her husband lived in Cleveland. Every Friday night, Susan raced out of the office to catch the 5:30 flight to Cleveland and every Sunday night she would take the last flight home to New Jersey. Pressed for time, Susan stopped exercising and was unable to stay on her diet.

After hearing about Susan's hectic schedule, I was not at all surprised to see that her blood pressure was going up, up, up. Having been so successful before in treating her high blood pressure herself, Susan was reluctant to take medication and I agreed with her. If possible, it is better to treat the cause of the problem than merely to treat the symptoms. So here's what we decided. If Susan was to maintain her health, she would have to change her lifestyle. In the long run, that meant that her husband would have to move to New Jersey, or she would find a job in Cleveland. In the short run, it meant sharing the stressful weekend commute with her husband so that he would visit her every other weekend. Susan also agreed to go back on her diet and exercise program. And finally, she promised to steer clear of airplane food, which is packed with salt and could be aggravating her high blood pressure. Within three months, her blood pressure was back to normal.

Often, changes in diet and lifestyle can have a positive effect on blood pressure. People who lose weight almost always drop a few points off their blood pressure and the same is true for people who exercise on a regular basis. Adding fiber, fresh fruits, and vegetables to your diet, which are high in potassium, can also help reduce blood pressure in many people. Cutting back on salt sometimes helps, and I'll talk about that later. I have also found that people who learn stress control techniques, such as biofeedback, meditation, or self-hypnosis, can also fare very well without drugs. Since I am not an expert on stress management, I refer these patients to a psychiatrist with whom I work closely.

When I have a patient with borderline hypertension and no other risk factors, I usually prescribe a nonmedical approach to treat her high blood pressure. Then, I monitor her very carefully, meaning that I will examine her weekly if I feel that her lifestyle or occupation puts her under unusual stress. In most cases, however, I follow up with the patient every three to six months.

If the patient has other risk factors, such as high cholesterol or elevated triglycerides, I don't take any chances—in terms of stroke and CAD, this combination can be deadly. In addition to recommending sensible lifestyle changes, I also include drug therapy to make sure the blood pressure returns to a normal level as soon as possible.

There are four major categories of medication for high blood pressure. Not all are appropriate for all patients; therefore, the physician must select the one that is best suited to the individual. Writing a prescription to lower blood pressure is only half the battle: The patient must be monitored very carefully to make sure that the medication is working properly and to watch for any undesirable side effects.

Diuretics

Diuretics cause the body to excrete excess salt and water, thus reducing the blood volume, the amount of fluid being pumped throughout the body.

When this happens, the heart doesn't have to work as hard and the blood pressure falls. These relatively inexpensive medications have been used since the 1950s to control hypertension. Commonly prescribed diuretics include Diuril, Lasix, and Hygroton. Diuretics used to be the first-choice drug to treat hypertension, but this is changing with the availability of other newer drugs.

Recent studies show that diuretics may cause higher cholesterol and blood sugar levels, actually increasing the risk for diabetes, heart attack, and stroke. In the process of eliminating salt and water, diuretics can also wash too much potassium out of the body, leaving the patient feeling dragged out and exhausted. In rare cases, they can cause stomach irritation, ulcers of the stomach and gastrointestinal tract, and even gout. Despite the negative side effects, diuretics are still very effective in the treatment of high blood pressure for many patients. Anyone taking this drug should have a blood lipid profile taken annually and should be carefully watched for low potassium levels or digestive disorders.

Beta Blockers

The sympathetic nervous system produces chemicals like adrenaline—the "fight or flight" hormone—that can make the arteries constrict, the heart beat more forcefully, and the blood pressure soar. Beta blockers interfere with the way these chemicals affect the heart and arteries, preventing the constriction of the small arteries that control blood pressure, the arterioles. Commonly prescribed beta blockers include Inderal, Timolol, and Lopressor. These drugs also reduce anxiety in many patients. Therefore, I often use beta blockers on extremely nervous or high-strung patients whom I feel could use a little calming down.

However, there are some potentially serious side effects. Some patients may become sluggish and depressed on these drugs and may feel too slowed down. Studies show that some men become impotent on beta blockers and that some women on these drugs may have difficulty achieving orgasm. One of the few studies of beta blockers to include women concluded that women may develop more complications on these drugs than men.

Finding the appropriate dose is critical. There is always a danger that if the heart is slowed down too much, the patient will feel constantly exhausted by the slightest exertion. And finally, in rare cases, the conduction of the heart rhythm may be so impaired that the impulse no longer passes from the upper to the lower chambers of the heart: This is called heart block, and if an effective and rapid enough "rescue rhythm" doesn't emerge to pace the heart, the situation is very serious. Anyone taking a beta blocker should be carefully monitored by her physician.

Angiotensin Inhibitors

Often, in the human body, one reaction triggers another and then another, and an entire chain of events depends on the presence of a certain chemical or enzyme. The following is a case in point. Angiotensin-converting enzyme (ACE) changes a substance called angiotensin into another compound that raises blood pressure by causing the smooth muscle cells of the blood vessels to constrict or narrow. The class of drugs called ACE inhibitors blocks this reaction. Therefore, the compound is not produced, the arteries don't constrict, and the blood pressure doesn't rise. This sounds terrific—and these drugs are terrific. For many patients, particularly African-Americans, they seem to work wonders.

In some patients, though, ACE inhibitors can cause unpleasant side effects. On rare occasions, a patient will develop an allergic reaction that produces swelling of the lips, throat, hands, and feet. Others get skin rashes, some so severe that they develop into a life-threatening illness called Stevens-Johnson syndrome. I am very careful when trying this type of medication (or any new drug) on highly allergic people. But for many other patients, ACE inhibitors are an excellent choice of medication and generally have fewer side effects than some of the other alternatives. Vasotec and Capoten are the most commonly prescribed ACE inhibitors.

Calcium Channel Blockers

The newest drugs on the block are relatively expensive, and although finding the right dose requires some skill on the part of the physician, many doctors— myself included—are very optimistic about this class of antihypertensives. As their name implies, calcium channel blockers have a direct effect on calcium. When calcium dissolved in the bloodstream is allowed to enter the muscle cells in arterial walls through special channels or pores in the cell membrane, it triggers events that cause the cell to shorten and the arteries to constrict or narrow. When this happens, the total capacity of the arteries is reduced, and if the total volume of blood remains constant, the blood pressure rises. The calcium channel blockers prevent the calcium from entering the cells: The "tone" in the wall of the arterioles is diminished, the vessels dilate, and the capacity expands. The blood pressure then falls.

Originally used to treat heart arrhythmias, calcium channel blockers have been only recently used to treat hypertension. The most commonly prescribed calcium channel blockers include the new long-acting Procardia XL, Cardizem, and Calan SR. Although they have fewer side effects than diuretics or beta blockers, in rare cases, they can cause heart block, rapid beating of the heart, or heart failure, and should also be monitored very carefully. Many physicians speculate that since women's arteries may be more prone to spasm than men's, calcium channel blockers, which relax the arteries, may work better on women than other medications. However, there is no hard evidence to back this up.

Diet

In the 1940s, before the widespread availability of medication to control high blood pressure, people with serious hypertension had only one treatment option, and it wasn't very pleasant: a drastically salt-reduced, low-calorie "rice diet," which was every bit as unappetizing as it sounds. Back then, the only thing we knew for certain about treating hypertension was that some people could significantly lower their blood pressure by avoiding salt. Now that we have other treatments, we no longer have to recommend such a stringent diet. And we now know for many patients it may have done more harm than good.

We also know that although salt can sometimes send blood pressure soaring, some people can use the salt shaker to their heart's content and still have normal blood pressure. The more we learn about the relationship between salt and high blood pressure, the more we see that there are no simple answers.

Salt, composed mainly of sodium, is not a natural enemy. Rather, it is a basic component of blood. To keep the body functioning normally, a normal salt-to-water ratio must be maintained. Excess salt and water is excreted in urine. Most of you know this from personal experience. For example, if you eat a very salty meal, you may still be extremely thirsty long after you've finished eating. That's because your body needs the extra water to maintain the normal salt/water balance. So you drink more fluid and make more frequent trips to the bathroom. However, if your body has a tendency to retain water, your blood volume will increase. As a result, your heart will have to work harder to circulate the added fluid and your blood pressure will rise. For most people, an occasional salty meal is not going to create a blood pressure crisis. But if you continually bombard your body with excess salt, or if your body has a low salt tolerance to begin with, which I'll explain later, you could be headed for trouble.

It's not surprising that studies show that people in countries that use a great deal of salt in their cooking tend to have higher blood pressures than people in countries that use little salt. In fact, the Japanese, whose cuisine is among the saltiest in the world, also have the highest blood pressure; so do Americans. Interestingly enough, in the United States we take it for granted that blood pressure will rise as we age. But in countries with low per-capita salt intake, blood pressure does not rise significantly after puberty. For example, blacks in

Africa, who typically eat a low-salt, high-fiber diet, have relatively low blood pressure, but for African-Americans, just the opposite is true. Nearly 50 percent of all African-Americans have high blood pressure, often beginning early in life.

Since blood pressure tends to be lower in the nonindustrialized countries, some people say that it is the stress of modern civilization that is to blame for the epidemic of high blood pressure, not salt intake. Is our diet to blame? Yes and no. Although 20 percent of Americans have high blood pressure, 80 percent do not. We can only assume that they must be eating pretty much the same diet as the people who are hypertensive. In addition, several studies comparing salt intake among individuals did not conclusively prove that people who eat the most salt have the highest blood pressure. Nor do studies prove conclusively that all people will develop high blood pressure who are fed a high-salt diet. The fact of the matter is that some will and some won't.

So it's reasonable to conclude that not everyone will be affected adversely by salt. Researchers now believe that some people may have inherited a tendency for salt sensitivity: If their salt intake is too high, they may indeed develop high blood pressure. A recent study gives some added weight to this theory. Researchers examined the kidney function of a group of young adult children of parents with high blood pressure who had normal pressure themselves. The researchers found that these children had a tendency to retain salt. Are these young adults going to develop high blood pressure later in life? Possibly. The researchers suggested that the study group may have inherited the salt sensitivity trait from their parents, and whether or not they develop high blood pressure could depend on a wide variety of factors, including diet.

How do we know who is salt sensitive and who isn't? We don't. In fact, we're not even certain that everyone who has high blood pressure is actually salt sensitive. In my own practice, I've had patients who have responded well to low-salt diets, and I've had patients whose blood pressure didn't drop one point on similar salt restriction. As a rule, I still think it makes good sense for people with high blood pressure to reduce their salt intake as much as possible. They should watch what they eat and not add additional salt to their food. If a patient has high blood pressure, certain highly processed, overly salted foods should also be eliminated, such as frozen pizza, canned salted vegetables, meals from fast-food restaurants, and the like. In rare cases, I may put a patient on a severely salt-restricted diet if I believe that it would be beneficial, but I do not recommend it for all patients.

People with normal blood pressure can afford an occasional trip to a fast-food restaurant or the luxury of a frozen TV dinner, but I wouldn't recommend it too often. In addition to tons of salt, this type of food is often loaded with fat and cholesterol, which may eventually find its way to your arteries. You can live a lot better without it. Also, if you're a woman who is bothered by bloating or water retention prior to your menstrual period, reducing your salt intake may help alleviate these symptoms. Since we know that high blood pressure can be hereditary, if you have a close relative, such as a parent or a sibling, who is hypertensive I would also suggest that you carefully watch your salt intake. Get out of the habit of adding salt to your food, and try in general to avoid eating highly salted food. Keep in mind just about anything you buy in the grocery store—from canned soup to canned nuts—has added salt, unless otherwise indicated on the package. So even if you don't put one extra grain of salt on your food, you can rest assured that you're getting plenty of it anyway.

Do not place yourself on a severely low-salt diet without first checking with your doctor. A recent study suggests that in some people a drastically salt-reduced diet can raise triglycerides and paradoxically, in some cases, actually raise blood pressure. Granted, it was a small study involving only 27 young men, but even so, I think that it's a bad idea to do anything that will drastically alter your body chemistry unless you are under the close supervision of a physician.

Chapter 11

WHEN DOES
RISK BEGIN?

SINCE children typically don't get heart attacks, we don't think of CAD as a childhood problem. However, many researchers believe that the arteriosclerotic process begins decades before the coronary arteries become clogged with plaque, sometimes in children as young as three years old.

Autopsies of very small children who died of unrelated causes have shown the presence of fatty streaks in their aortas, the large artery that receives blood from the left ventricle and sends it to the rest of the body. A fatty streak is a flat lesion composed mostly of fat and connective tissue, and it is similar to the larger plaque lesions that appear decades later. These same fatty streaks have been found in the coronary arteries of most adolescents. By age twenty, everyone has them.

So are these fatty streaks omens of the arteriosclerosis yet to come? Yes and no. We're not sure about the significance of these fatty streaks in the aorta, because so far there has been no proven connection between these lesions and the bigger fibrous plaque lesions. The fatty streaks in the coronary arteries are another story. These streaks often crop up in identical locations as the sites where the fibrous plaque will begin to collect decades later. That is why many researchers believe that these early fat deposits are a precursor of the full-blown arteriosclerotic lesion.

There's a great deal we still don't know about fatty streaks and the onset of arteriosclerosis. One of the biggest mysteries is that young women appear to have more fatty streaks than young men, yet young men suffer from more CAD than young women. Someday, we may be able to answer these questions. For now, all we can say is that based on our best information, it appears that fatty streaks in the young will result in the clogged coronary arteries of the middle-aged and elderly.

Many researchers also believe that it may be possible to nip them in the bud. That is, through early intervention, proper diet, exercise, and elimination of other risk factors, it may be possible to prevent the fatty streak from becoming the fat-laden plaque lesion. Although we can't say for certain that this is true, I feel it warrants careful consideration. Therefore, as a mother and a physician, I feel it's important to treat the adolescent with an eye on the future. Even if the fatty streak theory turns out to be pure whimsy, there is enough hard evidence to show that many American adolescents have lifestyles that could seriously endanger their future health:

- Studies show that 30 percent of all teenagers smoke by the time they get to high school. The rate is higher among teenage girls than boys.
- About 15 percent of all American children have cholesterol levels higher than the 150 mg/dl recommended for children. Many have cholesterol levels higher than the 200 mg/dl recommended for adults.
- Approximately 5 percent of all children have dangerously high cholesterol or triglycerides due to an inherited group of disorders called familial hyperlipidemias, and many of them don't even know it.
- About 12 percent of all adolescents have high blood pressure, that is, levels that are in the ninetieth percentile for their age. In many cases, their blood pressure will keep rising throughout adulthood, putting them at greater risk for CAD and stroke. (Between ages thirteen and fifteen, 95 percent of all teenagers have blood pressures below 136/86. Between ages sixteen and eighteen, 95 percent have pressures below 142/92. Anything higher than these pressures is considered bona fide hypertension. Levels in the ninetieth percentile for age are considered moderately high blood pressure.)
- Obesity among teens is on the rise, especially among teenage girls. According to a survey of twelve- to seventeen-year-olds, there has been a 39 percent increase in obesity between 1963 and 1980. Obese adolescents are more likely to have high cholesterol, elevated triglycerides, low levels of HDL, high blood pressure, and diabetes.

TEENAGERS AND CHOLESTEROL

Given the typical teenager's diet and lifestyle, it is no wonder that so many kids are severely overweight. Study after study shows that even though adults are getting more concerned about exercise and fitness, this trend has not trickled down to their kids. Teenagers today are still eating too much of the wrong foods and doing too little of the right activities. A typical snack in a fast-food restaurant can add up to more than 1,000 calories, and it will not be burned up in front of the television set or shopping at the mall. An order of fries and a double cheeseburger washed down with a chocolate malt is packed with saturated fat that can raise blood cholesterol.

The third of all adolescents who smoke are already causing serious damage to their coronary arteries that they will have to pay for down the road. Teenagers who experiment with drugs, especially crack and cocaine, are naively putting themselves at risk for life-threatening arrhythmias and sudden death. When a famous athlete dies of a massive heart attack induced by cocaine, it becomes a major news story and everyone from his coach to his college buddies are shocked. But those of us who work in big metropolitan hospitals have seen it all before.

We do not have a comprehensive plan in this country to address what I believe is a crisis in adolescent healthcare. Given all we know about smoking, if 30 percent of all teenagers still think it's okay to light up, then somehow we're not reaching them. If most kids don't know the difference between a saturated fat and a polyunsaturated fat, or how to make healthy food choices, then we adults—including doctors—are not doing our jobs.

There are some people who may feel that adolescents are naturally obstinate and there is no point in trying to get them to modify their behavior—they'll never listen anyway. Studies show just the opposite: If preteens are given the right direction, they will follow it. A case in point is a special study that involved adolescents in an affluent New York suburb and a middle-class neighborhood in the Bronx. Both groups of kids had their cholesterols screened at school. Only 11 percent of the children had cholesterol levels below the 140-mg/dl level recommended for their age group!

Throughout the school year, the children were given information on good diet, the importance of physical activity, and the negative effects of smoking. A follow-up study five years later showed that the kids who participated in the study showed significant improvement: They had a decline in cholesterol, better eating habits, and a decrease in smoking. Other studies of adolescents in similar programs in Finland and Norway also showed positive results, including a dramatic decline in smoking. Studies such as these make me think that our kids are starved for information. There is a crying need for school-based programs that can provide adolescents with the facts they need to make good choices.

CHOLESTEROL TESTING FOR CHILDREN

Given the current controversy over cholesterol testing for adults, it seems unlikely that the medical community will reach a consensus about the testing of children. And that's a shame, because there are many children who could benefit from it. On this issue I'm a hardliner: I would like to see all children have a cholesterol test before adolescence. I think they deserve it, and as a parent, I made sure both my children had one. But I'm also realistic, and I know that this probably will not become part of medical protocol at least in this century. However, if we're not going to test everyone, I feel that it's critical that we at least test the children who are at greatest risk. I said earlier that about 5 percent of all children have inherited a tendency for hyper-lipidemia, elevated blood lipids that are caused by a glitch in the normal metabolism of fats. Somewhere along the line, an important enzyme is missing or an important step in the metabolic process goes awry. When this happens, the child is often at risk for the early onset of CAD and premature death.

The earlier these children are treated—either through dietary changes, medication, or both—the better the prognosis. But first, problems must be detected, and that's trickier than it sounds. Since we don't routinely check children's cholesterol, we must somehow find these at-risk children. Because of the hereditary nature of hyperlipidemia, any parent who has an extremely high cholesterol (in the upper ninety-fifth percentile) should make sure that his or her children are also checked. Don't wait for your doctor or your child's doctor to suggest it. In my experience, most of them overlook it because they somehow don't make the connection.

There are other children who I feel would also benefit from cholesterol testing either because of their lifestyle or other risk factors. In fact, based on studies of risk factors among the young, I have compiled the following guide-lines for parents to determine which kids should be tested. A child should have a cholesterol test if:

1. She has a mother who had a heart attack before age sixty or a father who had a heart attack before age fifty.
2. Either parent or a sibling has an unusually high cholesterol (in the top ninety-fifth percentile).
3. She has a grandparent who died prematurely of CAD.
4. She has a grandparent who had a stroke before age sixty-five.
5. She is a teenager on birth control pills.
6. She is a teenager who smokes.
7. She is obese, or 30 percent above her normal weight.
8. She is diabetic.
9. She has high blood pressure—that is, she has readings above the ninety-fifth percentile for her age.
10. She is extremely aggressive, hostile, or under a great deal of stress.

All children who have elevated cholesterol should also have blood lipid profiles to determine what, if any, treatment is necessary. About 15 to 20 percent of children with high cholesterol also have proportionately high levels of HDL, the good cholesterol, and are not considered high-risk. A thorough lipid profile will determine if there is a specific familial hyperlipidemia, that is, a particular genetic metabolic disorder.

Hyperlipidemia can only be diagnosed by the appropriate blood tests. It's not for a parent to decide that his or her child has a problem without consulting a physician. Nor should a parent impose a severely restrictive diet on a child unless it is under the supervision of a physician. Regardless of weight or cholesterol levels, children need a well-balanced diet to develop properly. Devising an eating plan for an overweight adolescent requires expert skill. Since adolescents especially are sensitive about their weight and eating habits, establishing a food plan for a teenager also requires a certain amount of finesse. I have found that teenagers often work better with a professional than they do with their own parents, so I usually refer my younger patients to a qualified nutritionist.

Under the age of two, cholesterol intake should not be restricted because children need the extra fat for normal brain development and to produce extra cells for growth. Mother Nature knew what she was doing when she put cholesterol in breast milk! After two years old, children with extremely high cholesterols may need to be on a low-fat diet.

Low-Risk Children

As I've said earlier, I think it's a good idea to know your child's cholesterol and I would certainly have my children tested at least once before the age of twelve. If everything is normal, repeat the test every five years. As far as diet is concerned, I feel that most everyone—men, women, and children—can benefit from the so-called prudent diet recommended by the American Heart Association. I think that everyone should restrict their intake of fat to 30 percent of their daily calories, with only 10 percent in the form of saturated fat. It is really not a hardship and still gives you tremendous leeway in terms of the types of food you can eat. For most people, minor dietary changes— switching from whole milk to skim milk, cutting back on meat in favor of a few fish meals a week, and adding fiber to breakfast cereal—may be all it takes to trim the fat from their diet.

Keep in mind that following a low-fat diet may not only help prevent coronary heart disease but other diseases as well, such as ovarian cancer, breast cancer, and colon cancer. We're not exactly sure why. One theory is that organic toxins like insecticides and food additives remain in the body stored in fat deposits and may contribute to the abnormal cell growth typical of cancer. In addition, an excess amount of body fat triggers hormonal changes that may also be responsible for certain types of cancer.

Critics may say that there is no concrete evidence that children raised on a nutritionally sound, low-fat diet will fare better than those raised on the traditional high-fat diet. This is true. It will probably be several decades before the diet hypothesis is proved or disproved to everyone's satisfaction. However, I feel that there is a good chance that a low-fat diet could prevent or delay the onset of arteriosclerosis, and as a mother, I want my children to have that advantage.

V

THE FEMALE HEART
AND THE FEMALE MIND

✣

Chapter 12

THE STRESSED-OUT WOMAN

WHEN I think of the devastating effect that stress can have on the heart and soul, I think of Brenda, a fifty-six-year-old friend and patient who is well aware that her lifestyle is slowly killing her. Much to my frustration, she believes that there is nothing she can do about it.

For the past four years, Brenda has had unstable high blood pressure that cannot be controlled by medication. When she is in my office talking about her life, the sphygmomanometer soars to 160/120 and I am afraid that it frequently rises to dangerous heights when she is angry or upset. To make matters worse, Brenda is one of my few patients who is still a chain smoker and refuses to stop because she says it offers the few moments of relaxation in her otherwise hectic life.

Neither Brenda's work nor home life is very satisfying. As personnel man-ager for a leading international advertising agency, her days are spent manag-ing a creative staff and a secretarial staff that are always at each other's throats. Her private life offers little relief from the daily tension. Divorced 15 years ago and recently remarried, Brenda has one son, Steve, a twenty-eight-year-old who has made a career out of graduate school. Since her ex-husband refuses to provide any support for Steve, he is constantly hitting Brenda for money, much to the chagrin of her second husband Don, who is always admonishing her for indulging him.

The owner of a small but moderately successful printing plant, Don is struggling to support two college-age children and a wife from a previous marriage. Don, who admittedly works extremely hard, would like to retire within ten years and is trying to accumulate a nest egg. He doesn't hide the fact that he is very annoyed that Brenda is unable to contribute equally to their retirement fund because she is still supporting her son. Although Don expects Brenda to split her paycheck, he is unwilling to split the housework. In fact, he expects Brenda to manage the household and do all the cooking even on the weekends when his children come to visit.

Although Brenda feels their arrangement is unfair—and I believe that she is furious about it—she doesn't complain because she simply assumes that Don is unwilling to change. Nor is she willing to confront her son about getting a job for fear of alienating him. As a result of all the turmoil in her life, Brenda is a seething mass of anger and rage, most of it turned against herself.

Brenda knows that she's in trouble and is deeply worried about her health. During her last office visit, her gray eyes filled with tears and she said sadly, "Marianne, my mother had a heart attack when she was sixty-eight and I'm afraid that my heart won't last even that long." With three major risk factors for CAD—smoking, high blood pressure, and acute stress—Brenda has a point, although I am not as pessimistic. I believe that Brenda has the power to alter her fate. However, in order for her to reduce her risk of heart attack, Brenda needs to learn to control the emotional problems I believe are at the root of her physical ones.

Brenda's case is hardly unusual. In fact, I would venture to guess that many doctors have a high percentage of patients with physical problems that are a direct result of lives filled with stress, anger, and unresolved conflicts.

Although the traditional medical school education still emphasizes the physical origins of illness, most doctors today recognize that there is a definite link between the body and the mind. As in Brenda's case, there are some ailments in which our usual cures offer little comfort, and therefore we must look for solutions outside of conventional medicine. But before we can talk about ways of preventing negative emotions from exacting a painful toll on our bodies, we must understand exactly how our feelings can affect our health. And in order to understand what stress does to the body, we must first understand a little bit about evolution—how human beings developed through the ages.

Our response to stress is regulated by the autonomic or involuntary nervous system, the same system that controls other vital functions including the beating of the heart. Similar to the beating of the heart—which requires no active intervention on our part—when we are confronted with a life-threatening or stressful situation our body responds automatically. The autonomic nervous system is divided into two parts: the sympathetic nervous system and the parasympathetic nervous system, or the vagal system. For some unknown reason, a small minority of people are vagal responders, that is, when they are under stress the parasympathetic nervous system takes over. Their blood pressure suddenly plunges, their heart rate drops, and often they faint. Although this reaction may be inconvenient at times and downright embarrassing, it is not life-threatening. In fact, within a few minutes the vagal responder should be back to normal.

Most people, however, respond to stress through the sympathetic nervous system that regulates the more typical flight or fight response, a defense mechanism scientists believe originated millions of years ago to accommodate the lifestyle of our primitive ancestors. When the cortex of the brain perceives a threat, it signals the sympathetic nervous system to generate a series of physiologic responses that tells the body to gear up for action. The adrenal glands begin to pump higher quantities of catecholamines—epinephrine and norepinephrine—that in turn trigger a chain of reactions. The kidneys release renin, which raises the blood pressure and forces the heart to pump faster. They also hold on to salt and water to increase the blood volume in case of injury. The digestive system stops abruptly as blood flows away from the stomach to the skeletal muscles in preparation for physical activity. The body consumes more oxygen to fuel these changes. The pupils dilate, allowing more light to enter the eye for better night vision. We are ready to fight for our lives, or to flee for our survival.

In the days of cave life, we would have followed through with the appropriate burst of physical activity, and within a few minutes our bodies would have returned to normal. However, modern men and women do not live in caves—we live in bustling cities and sprawling suburbs where we sit behind desks in modern office buildings or tend to our families in ranch-style houses. Although we don't spend our days hunting or being hunted, life is not carefree. We still encounter stress at work, at home, and in our personal relationships and we still respond to it much the same way as our ancestors did. Our sympathetic nervous system doesn't differentiate between fear generated by a wild animal on the rampage or rage directed at a spouse. Strong emotions such as anger, frustration, hostility, and sometimes even depression can be perceived as threatening enough to trigger the primitive flight or fight response. Most of the time we don't fight or flee: We sit and simmer and turn our anger inward.

Our highly sensitive sympathetic nervous system may have helped keep our ancestors safe from harm, but for some of us the physiologic responses that shift the body into high gear can be deadly. For some people, the flight or fight reaction can send an unstable heart into a lethal arrhythmia, seriously elevate blood pressure, impair the flow of oxygen to the heart, and even destroy heart muscle. Some studies suggest that surges of catecholamines may actually cause injury to arteries, thus promoting arteriosclerosis.

Voodoo death is a dramatic example of how stress—or actually fear—can kill, not by black magic but by disrupting normal heart rhythms. At the turn of the century, a renowned medical researcher, Walter Cannon of Harvard, first theorized that voodoo death was not caused by supernatural powers but was actually a result of a series of sympathetic nervous system discharges that resulted in ventricular fibrillation, a lethal arrhythmia. In other words, the victims of so-called voodoo death had been literally scared to death by the mere belief that the voodoo practitioners had some mystical power over them.

Since then, other studies have proven Cannon's hypothesis that anxiety can affect the heart's natural rhythm.

Although few of us have to worry about being targeted by voodoo priests or encountering an equally terrifying situation, our lives are hardly anxiety-free. For some people, even moderate amounts of anxiety are enough to cause cardiac abnormalities. A case in point is a common situation: driving in heavy traffic. A recent study used portable or Holter monitors to compare the heart rates of 24 patients with CAD with 32 normal cardiac patients as the participants drove through traffic-jammed streets. Three of the normal patients developed abnormalities in their electrocardiogram (EKG), showing signs of oxygen deprivation and strain. All of the 24 cardiac patients experienced an increase in heart rate—some soaring to 140 beats per minute—and their abnormal EKG became even more abnormal. Five developed extra ventricular beats, which could develop into a potentially dangerous arrhythmia.

Another study measured the effect of public speaking on the heart. At a recent medical meeting, 23 cardiac-normal physicians and 7 diagnosed with CAD were put on Holter monitors as they delivered a speech before their peers. Six of the so-called normal doctors developed extra ventricular beats and six of the seven doctors with CAD developed signs of ischemia or oxygen deprivation. Five of the CAD patients developed arrhythmias.

From these studies we can see that routine, daily stress can exact its toll on both healthy and unhealthy hearts. This is not to say, however, that we are putting our life on the line every time we encounter a stressful situation; or, that every time you sit in traffic, speak in public, or even argue with your spouse you are putting yourself at risk of having a heart attack or developing a life-threatening arrhythmia. If this were the case, no one would survive to adulthood because life is filled with stress. Fortunately, we are able to cope with the peaks and valleys of daily life by finding constructive outlets for our frustration and anger.

Sometimes circumstances can arise that can throw even the most well-balanced person into the kind of emotional turmoil that can literally make her sick. Studies show that people who may be prone to heart attacks are those who have experienced repeated bouts of stress from many sources. There are times when we all may encounter periods of intense stress. Divorce, death of a spouse or a parent, difficulty with a child, loss of a job, or even an unexpected financial reversal are commonplace events that can generate uncommon amounts of stress. Any severe emotional blow can have a devastating effect on health. Therefore, I feel that during periods of crises or acute unhappiness it is critical to get outside help. I often refer my patients to a psychiatrist with whom I work closely for short-term therapy. At times, I also refer them for marriage or family counseling if I feel it will help them better cope with a difficult home environment. Psychological counseling is not just for "sick" people. It is for anyone who is under a great deal of stress and may need assistance through a stormy period.

THE STRESS–PRONE PERSONALITY

There are some people who appear to be more stress-sensitive than others, and as a result they are more prone to experience lethal reactions. Some of them may have a nervous system that is more vulnerable to emotional swings, switching into high gear with little provocation. Some may have a personality that "takes everything to heart," experiencing more emotional tumult than the average person.

Similar to other medical research, the original research done on personality, stress, and heart disease was very male-oriented. The profile that emerged of the coronary-prone individual was of a middle-aged man with what was dubbed type A personality. Typically, Mr. Type A (although some women were included in the profile, it was predominantly male) is a driven, compulsive workaholic who is consumed by his job. Mr. Type A worries a lot about everything, especially the office, where he feels responsible for his job and everyone else's. He is poor at delegating work and rarely takes a vacation. According to researchers Rosenman and Friedman who first coined the term *type* A, this individual is impatient to achieve what are usually poorly defined goals: He wants to get rich quick, or become president of the company, but he doesn't understand the steps he needs to take to make his dreams come true. In sum, Mr. Type A is a difficult, single-minded, one-dimensional person who is exactly the kind of man you don't want to marry. If you are married to one, however, be sure he is well insured: Type A men are said to have 1.7 to 4.5 times the rate of CAD as compared to their nicer, more even-tempered type B counterparts.

The Framingham study also noted an increased risk of CAD among type A men, but interestingly enough, found an increased risk of heart disease among type B, or passive, women married to overly demanding type A men. According to Framingham, whether you are male or female, high levels of hostility and unexpressed anger can increase your risk of having a heart attack.

The concept of the type A personality has been challenged by studies such as the famous Mr. Fit Trials, which did not find a significant correlation between personality and heart attack. To this day, researchers are still arguing over whether personality plays any role at all in the onset of heart disease for either men or women. I believe that it does, especially for women with a chronically stressful life. Based on my personal experiences with women patients, I have identified six types of women who I feel are at the greatest risk of ending up as cardiac patients.

Type A for Anger

As we have seen, chronic hostility and anger keeps the central nervous system pumping chemicals that can actually cause damage to vital arteries. Whereas a type A man may show the outward manifestations of aggression—he'll be combative at the slightest provocation or he'll show his impatience if he feels that someone isn't performing a task fast enough for him—the type A woman often does a better job of hiding her anger and frustration. Since it is not socially acceptable for women to rant and rave, the angry woman learns to smile on the outside although she is seething on the inside.

Typically, hostile women are involved in relationships over which they feel they have no control. When I think of classic type A women, two patients come to mind. The first is a woman with high blood pressure who is married to a chronic "womanizer" who has chased other women throughout their 20-year marriage. Although she is furious at her husband, she doesn't feel that there is anything she can do to alter his behavior. The second is a successful, overachieving executive who is spending her life seeking her mother's approval. Her mother is a demanding, selfish woman who is simply not capable of giving the kind of uncritical love that her daughter is seeking. Unless these women find a way to defuse their anger, their health is in serious jeopardy.

The Nice Girl

She's just the girl who can't say no . . . to her colleagues, her boss, her husband, or her children. This woman wants to be liked and admired, and as a result she tries to do ten times more than is humanly possible. She'll offer to cater single-handedly her mother-in-law's birthday party even though it coincides with her busiest week at the office. She'll agree to run the church fund-raising bazaar even though the burden falls on her every year. She'll stay up half the night baking homemade cookies for her daughter's Christmas party at school instead of buying them at a bakery, because she doesn't feel that her child should have to make any compromises just because her mother works. The nice girl is well liked, but she is paying a steep price for her popularity. She is placing herself under too much stress, which is definitely not good for her heart or her health. If she continues to devote her life to pleasing others, she will eventually become infuriated, with herself and with the other people in her life. When the nice girl gets fed up, she could be transformed into the angry woman.

The Doormat

Unlike the nice girl, the submissive woman doesn't have an overwhelming desire to please. A combination of circumstance and a passive nature has put her in a subordinate role, either at work, or at home, or both. No matter what kind of relationship this woman enters into, she manages to feel as if she is getting shortchanged, and often she is. The doormat probably has a low-paying but highly demanding job. She is the woman who sits at a switchboard eight hours a day, and has to make elaborate arrangements to find someone to fill in for her every time she has to go to the bathroom. She is the woman who is packed up to go home at 5:30 P.M. on a Friday only to have her boss suddenly dump ten letters on her desk that must go out immediately. Her boss goes to his country home, while she stays late finishing the work. This woman has little control over her job and probably even less control over her life. To compound her problem, her husband may be unsympathetic and overly demanding. Dissatisfied with most aspects of her life, this woman is frustrated and unhappy, and although she may be unaware of it, she has a lot of hidden hostility.

The Neglected Caregiver

She's the woman who takes care of everybody else, but forgets to do even the most fundamental things for herself. She'll make sure that her children and her husband get their annual physicals, but her visits to the doctor are typically sporadic. Her days revolve around caring for others and that is how she derives her self-worth and satisfaction. Although this woman appears to be motivated by concern for others, I believe that her true motivation is fear. Deep down, she feels unworthy of attention. She is terrified at the thought of being scrutinized and judged, and therefore she hides behind other people, making their lives her life. Because they neglect their health, these women are at greater risk of developing heart disease than women who take even moderately good care of themselves. To compound the problem, since caregivers are reluctant to ask for help for themselves, they are more likely to ignore chest pain or other early warning signs of heart attack or CAD.

The Overloaded Woman

She is the woman who is juggling two or three jobs simultaneously: working in the home, working outside of the home, and maybe even helping to care for an elderly relative in somebody else's home. In all likelihood, she is not only a breadwinner but is largely responsible for raising the kids and running the household. Not surprisingly, most of the time the overloaded woman is exhausted. She has neither the time nor the energy to exercise, and very likely she is not as careful about her diet as she should be.

Her body is continually under stress, and that is not good for either her heart or her soul. Some studies suggest that women who literally go from their day job to their night job with no break in between may show signs of physical strain. According to one study done by Dr. Marianne Frankenhauser at the University of Stockholm, men and women have markedly different physical responses to the end of the workday. When men get home from work, they begin to "unwind": Their blood pressure drops and the levels of catecholamines drop too. According to the study, women stay "switched on" until much later in the evening, as demonstrated by their elevated blood pressure and high levels of catecholamines. My guess is that most women don't really get a chance to kick off their shoes and put up their feet until the last child is sound asleep, as reflected in their cardiovascular response.

The overloaded woman has another problem: Wherever she is and whatever she is doing she has a nagging feeling that she should be doing something else. At work, she thinks about home. At home, she thinks about work. As a result, she doesn't feel that she is doing either job very well, and this too can be very stressful.

The Isolated Woman

Studies show that people living in social isolation are more prone to illness and death than those who are socially connected. Typically, widowed people have higher rates of illness—including heart disease—and die younger than those who still have mates. More women will end up living alone than men. Between ages fifty-five and sixty-four, one out of five women will lose their husbands. Since women typically outlive men, there is a four out of five chance that a woman will end up alone. Although living alone should not be synonymous with isolation, in reality it often is, especially for a woman who is accustomed to being part of a family and a marriage. In order to protect her health, the isolated woman needs to learn how to reach out to others and to build a new life.

TRYING TO CHANGE

Although these women appear to have very different problems, they share one common link: None of them have learned how to take care of themselves in a healthfully selfish manner. In her ground-breaking book, A *Different Voice*, psychologist Carol Gilligan noted that women cannot develop self-esteem until they recognize that their own needs are as important as everybody else's. I would go even further and say that women cannot be truly healthy until they learn how to care for themselves at least as well as they care for everybody else.

More often than not, women neglect their own emotional and physical needs. They give much and expect little in return. As a result, many go through life feeling angry and cheated, often paying a steep price in terms of their own personal health. In extreme cases, an angry, hostile woman who does not confront her feelings openly often expresses them in terms of a wide range of physical ailments including ulcers, heart palpitations, insomnia, and chest pain. However, even women who are not raging on the inside may be at risk if their lives are totally focused on others. If a woman's life revolves around meeting the needs of others, she is more likely than not to neglect her own needs. I believe that a woman who is so out of touch with her own emotional needs is less likely to acknowledge physical symptoms, such as chest pain, and more likely to suffer a heart attack in silence.

When I see a woman in my practice who I feel is under a great deal of stress, I encourage her to take stock of her life so she can identify the source of her anxiety. I ask her to divide her life into three main components: personal relationships, work, and solitary pleasures. We then discuss what portion of her time and emotional energy is consumed by each of these categories. Ideally, life should be a balance between these three often opposing forces, but usually it is not. Women are typically laden with family and work responsibilities, leaving little time left for themselves. I then have to convince my patient that she needs to make some constructive changes in her lifestyle.

Solitary Pleasures

Every woman has to have some sense of herself outside of her family or marriage. All too often, a woman's identity becomes merged with her husband's or her children's. It's critical for a woman to maintain a piece of her life just for herself. Try to devote a portion of your day to pursuing a personal interest that is all your own: Find a hobby, preferably one that puts you in touch with other people. Take up a sport such as tennis or golf that can help you create a social network outside of your family. If hobbies don't interest you, join a book discussion group, or adopt a cause in which you can donate your time and meet people with similar interests. Maintaining a separate existence will give you a sense of self-confidence that can be a great source of security.

Every woman also needs a place that is just for her, preferably where she can shut the door and have some privacy. It's important for family members to know that you are not on call 24 hours a day. If you don't have an extra room, stake out a corner of the basement or convert a utility closet into a tiny study. At the very least, create a small reading area for yourself in your bedroom.

Every woman needs to incorporate some form of regular exercise into her life. Exercise is a terrific stress buster. Moderately strenuous exercise requires physical and mental concentration. For most people, anxious thoughts seem to vanish when they're in the middle of a vigorous workout, a game of tennis, or a brisk walk through the park. Exercise also provides a healthy outlet for the fight or flight response. The catecholamines discharged by the sympathetic nervous system that prepare our bodies for activity are put to good use when we engage in physical activity.

Exercise is also a proven mood enhancer. If we exercise long enough, our bodies begin to produce certain chemicals called endorphins that actually make us feel better. That is why most people feel relaxed and invigorated after a good workout. I know that most women's lives are laden with responsibility, but never forget that your first responsibility is to your own health. If you are not exercising on a regular basis, find the time to do so. Get up a half hour earlier in the morning to take a walk, enroll in a dance class during lunch, or go swimming after work. No matter how you do it, make sure that you get enough physical activity. If you do, you will find that you are better equipped to deal with your other responsibilities.

Every woman also needs to have some downtime in her life. Ever since my children were very small, I have gotten up an hour earlier every day so I can have a cup of coffee in peace and think about the day ahead before anyone else gets to the breakfast table. I jealously guard this hour of private reflection and will forego it only if an emergency arises in my family or in my practice. If you can find a half hour of private time during the day to unwind, you will reap the benefits for the rest of the day.

I can certainly sympathize with a woman whose time is rarely her own, but I really do believe that if you can't find at least an hour a day to do something for yourself, you must be doing something wrong. Can anyone else in your household assume some of your responsibilities? Can you hire someone to help with cleaning or babysitting? Does your community center offer resources, such as babysitting or assistance in caring for an elderly relative, of which you are not taking advantage?

Very often, women mistakenly assume that there is no one around who is willing or able to help them. A case in point is my patient Ann, a legal secretary who confessed that she dreaded her upcoming vacation because she was going to spend it taking her ailing mother to an assortment of medical specialists. I nodded sympathetically and then began to think that it was a ridiculous way for her to spend one of her two precious vacation weeks. I asked her if there was anyone else who could escort her mother so that Ann could at least go away for a few days. At first, she was emphatic that there was no one around who could help, and not only that but her mother would not want to accept help from anyone else. I then began to ask her a few questions about her life, including whether or not she belonged to any particular religious organizations. Ann's face brightened and she replied that her family had close ties with the local church. In fact, the pastor had called her last week to see how her mother was doing and to ask if she needed any help. Ann said that she had dismissed his offer because she didn't want to bother anybody with her problems. I convinced Ann to call him back to see if he could find some volunteers who could help her during her week off.

Ann's pastor found half a dozen parishioners who knew her family well and were more than happy to lend a hand. Much to Ann's surprise, her mother was pleased with the arrangement because it gave her an opportunity to become reacquainted with old friends. The moral of this story is a simple one: We often neglect to tap valuable resources because we are uncomfortable about accepting help. If you find that you are unable to find any free time in your schedule, then it's time to look for the potential untapped resources in your life.

Personal Relationships

When I encounter a woman who I feel is consumed with anger, I try to help her focus on her own personal needs. I start off by asking her a simple question that many women have difficulty answering: "Just exactly what do you require from your relationships to be happy?" Frequently, these women are startled by the question—they do not think of personal relationships as something over which they have any control. What they don't realize is that we have enormous control over our relationships. In fact, we create them simply by how we view ourselves, and how we present ourselves to others. If we believe that we are worthwhile, important people deserving of love and respect, in most cases, we will command it from those with whom we come in contact. If we are willing to endure disrespect and inconsiderate treatment, in many cases, that is what we will get. This is not to say that every relationship will be equal, or that we will always get out what we put in. Sometimes we are called upon to make sacrifices and to give more than we will receive. But it should never be the case all the time, and if it is, it is a sign of an unhealthy pattern.

Demanding a certain level of reciprocity in our relationships is not only good for us but good for the other important people in our life. If we are not properly loved or cared for, we will not be able to love or care properly for those who need us. If a woman continually feels as if her spouse is taking advantage of her, she may go through the motions of being a wife, but she quietly seeks revenge by holding back in countless other ways. If a woman feels that her children are overly demanding and underappreciative, she may give in to their constant demands, but she feels resentful when she does. If a woman feels that she is always there for her friends when they need her, but they vanish when she is in need, she may feel she is being used. In every relationship, there is an unspoken personal contract that dictates the way we relate to each other. If we feel that we are continually giving of ourselves and not getting anything in return, it's time to change the rules. Granted, it is usually not easy to do, and that is why I often refer patients in this predicament to a professional such as a therapist or marriage counselor. Often, the whole family can benefit from counseling.

Sometimes, however, renegotiating a relationship is not possible without destroying it. If you want to remain a part of it without destroying your health, you have to let go of your anger. Take my patient, Susan, who after 16 years of marriage and raising two children resumed her career as a teacher. Although Susan had run the household single-handedly for years, after she went back to work she expected her husband to take over some of the tasks. Her husband, however, was extremely reluctant to assume new responsibilities. Not only did he work long hours running his own small jewelry business but he honestly believed his wife's first obligation was to be a mother, homemaker, and social director. Susan was furious about what she viewed as his stubbornness, and he was angry with her for changing the rules midgame.

The deadlock was finally broken when during a heart-to-heart talk I devised a practical solution. I advised Susan to sit down and take inventory of everything she was getting from her husband. When she actually focused on the overall relationship, she grudgingly admitted that her husband had a number of good qualities: He was faithful, a considerate lover, a good breadwinner, a wonderful father, attentive to her elderly parents, and never forgot an important birthday or anniversary. Susan conceded that even though he was not supportive about housework, in his own way her husband was contributing a great deal to the relationship. Only then was she able to overcome her anger and continue her marriage without jeopardizing her health. If her balance sheet had come up short on his end, the story could have had quite a different ending. Although I believe in doing all you can to preserve a good relationship, I have supported a patient's decision to leave a toxic relationship. Quite often, however, simply getting a patient to air her grievances can have a salutary effect on the relationship and her health.

Healthy relationships with people who we care about and who care about us are as important to our survival as food and water. In fact, studies show that people who lack this kind of companionship get sick more often and die younger than those who don't. In some respects, the woman who travels solo is at a disadvantage. Women who are married with families usually have a built-in social network at their disposal, but women who live alone often have a tougher job cultivating friendships and forming relationships. Nevertheless, their lives can be every bit as rich as women with partners, but it does take extra effort.

Today, more and more women are living alone for longer periods of time. Some women choose to postpone marriage until they are established in their careers; others live alone due to divorce or widowhood. As a woman who has been divorced for more years than I have been married, and who has had to face the challenge of making a new life for myself, I understand both the pitfalls and advantages of living alone.

When you live alone, you don't have to accommodate anyone else's schedule or desires. You can eat, sleep, or work any time you want. You can spend your money any way you choose as long as the monthly bills are covered. Basically, your only responsibility is to yourself. As a result of all of this autonomy, many women do the best work in their career during the times they live alone. There are women who live alone and simply love it, but there are also many women who do not live alone by choice.

Through the eyes of many women in my practice, I have watched husbands fall ill and die, grown children move out, and friends grow old or move on. Some of these women wither away before my eyes, becoming entombed in sadness, loneliness, and isolation. Other women, however, not only survive these losses but demonstrate remarkable resilience. Of course, even these women experience painful and difficult times adjusting to being no longer part of a couple or no longer at the hub of a busy family, but when they emerge from their grief their life is far from over.

I have observed one striking difference between the women who keep going and those who give up: The women who overcome the sorrow of loss are those who have the strongest sense of themselves. Typically, these survivors have managed to maintain a separate identity outside of their families. Their self-worth is not derived solely from taking care of others or living vicariously through others. These women don't necessarily have fabulous careers or even fascinating hobbies. In fact, many have devoted their lives to homemaking and raising their children, but in the process they did not forget to set aside some personal time to pursue their own interests and maintain their own friendships. Even though these women may feel their grief every bit as intensely as those who did not maintain a separate identity, they have other resources to fall back on to help fill the void.

Creating a new life for yourself is not easy and often the woman alone encounters her share of rejection. Many people do not socialize with women unless they are part of a couple: Perhaps a young, single woman is too threatening; perhaps the sight of a woman alone is too frightening to those who feel tenuous about their own relationships. Sadly, there are single women who fall into this archaic way of thinking. For instance, one of my patients, a recent widow who loves to entertain, said she was reluctant to give a dinner party because she didn't know any single men who could be her date. "Who wants to feel like a fifth wheel?" she asked. As a single woman who entertains a great deal myself, I chided her for being so narrow-minded. I reminded her that there is no law that states that there must be equal numbers of men and women at every social function nor do couples need only to socialize with other couples from similar backgrounds. In fact, some of the most memorable parties I have given were those in which I mixed married couples with single people, and older people with younger ones. As long as people are interesting and have something to talk about, they don't need to have a lot in common to enjoy each other's company, at least for the duration of one dinner party.

So if you like to entertain, reach out to people and invite them to your home whether or not you have a man around to play the role of host. Think of reasons to do this: Is there a friend celebrating a particular achievement? Give him a dinner party. Has one of your friends just come back from an important trip? Ask her and a few others to lunch to hear what tales she brings from other parts of the world. Call up one of your siblings you haven't seen in a long time. Family reminiscences can be particularly strengthening and rewarding to share. They remind you that, in fact, you are part of a social unit with a common history.

Don't keep track of who returns your invitation and who doesn't—it is irrelevant. You are not entertaining the people you like and love for a return engagement; you are planning festivities for your own enjoyment! Your job is to make sure that you have the comfort and stimulation of meaningful human contact, and as long as your needs are being met, don't keep a social score card.

It is also your responsibility to make sure that your need for physical warmth is being met—sexual and otherwise. Everyone needs the comfort of a caress, the reassurance of a hug, or even the feel of a warm handshake. From our earliest days of life, love and approval are expressed in terms of hugging, kissing, or a reassuring pat. Just because a spouse dies or you get divorced doesn't mean you should do without this source of great comfort. Hug your friends, cuddle your grandchildren, and get a pet you can kiss and hold.

Just because you may be older, don't rule out the possibility of romantic relationships. As a woman ages, the pool of available men dwindles, and I have seen women so discouraged by the statistics that they give up before they get started. They see themselves as old and undesirable, and therefore they opt out of the romantic arena. Although our culture equates youth with attractiveness, studies show that sexual interest is more based on finding a kindred spirit than on age or beauty. Interestingly enough, the women I know who see themselves as sexy, desirable people who have something to offer inevitably find a mate.

To a woman alone, the world can sometimes appear to be a cold, cruel place. Not everyone is going to be accepting of you, and at times you may reach out only to be rejected. But don't blame every rejection on the fact that you are alone or female or old. As I tell my patients, everyone—whether they are married, single, widowed, divorced, male or female—suffers from rejection at one time or another. If you succeed one out of ten times in whatever endeavor you are pursuing, you're well ahead of the game.

Women who are alone must be very careful not to fixate on what they lack;

they should focus on what they've still got. When I encounter a single woman who is questioning her self-worth, I advise her to sit down and make a list of her achievements. If she is still a size 12 or under, I tell her to write it down. If she is a terrific mother or a respected professional or both, I tell her to write it down. If she is a great dancer or a wiz with a tennis racket or a golf club, I tell her to write it down. If she devotes time to helping others or is a terrific cook, I tell her to write it down. By the end of the exercise, most women are quite surprised to see that they have accomplished a great deal more than they usually give themselves credit for and the realization can be a major ego booster.

For women who have been isolated, the idea of starting over may be overwhelming. The longer you remain out of the mainstream, the harder it is to get back. Often, loneliness feeds on itself: If you are depressed and isolated, your interpersonal skills may get rusty, and inadvertently you may actually push people away. Keep in mind that most everyone responds to a warm, friendly smile.

After a particularly difficult time in my own life, I felt that I needed to relearn how to be with others in social situations. I began by practicing on people who waited on me in stores. I tried to be aware of them as people, to ask them questions about themselves, and to thank them or make them feel appreciated if they had waited on me carefully or with particular thoughtfulness. It was a wonderful exercise. I began to experience shopping as a way to reenter social relationships and marveled to see how people unfolded and flowered with just a little attention and appreciation. Many of them had important and useful things to say. I learned an invaluable lesson from this experience: If people feel that you are genuinely happy to see them, they will in all likelihood feel the same way about you.

It's also important to remember that you don't have to be a brilliant intellectual to engage someone else in conversation. If you keep current and are interested in life, other people will find you interesting. If you are truly concerned about other people and ask them about themselves in an interested way, chances are that they will be more than happy to talk to you. In short, try to take the focus off yourself—how awkward you feel, how old you are, whether or not your wrinkles show—and put it on the other person.

The woman alone may have to reach out and extend herself in a special way to ensure that she has a full, meaningful life, but the rewards can be great in terms of personal satisfaction and good health.

The Workplace

Some women work because they have to. Some women work because they want to. And other women work for both the psychological and emotional income. Whether a woman jumps out of bed every morning eager to go to work, or develops stomach pains at the mere thought of her job, she must cope with her share of stress in the workplace.

No job is stress-free, and even the best of jobs are at times anxiety-provoking. However, the best of jobs are not evenly divided between men and women. On average, women earn substantially less than men and are more likely to be in dead-end, often boring jobs. Women are also more likely to be in subordinate roles, often having to report to several bosses. Even if the work is a bit dull at times and the pay is less than generous, most women can tolerate their jobs as long as they feel that they are treated with respect by their superiors and co-workers. Studies show that women who are the most unhappy at work are those who feel that they are not respected by their bosses and that they are treated as something less than human. Why do they stay in jobs they hate? The main reason is they don't believe they can do any better.

Any woman who finds herself in this situation is going to be constantly angry and frustrated. In order to preserve both her physical and emotional health, she needs to change her working conditions or to change her job. Very often, this kind of woman requires counseling to help her learn how to renegotiate her "contract" with her boss. Short-term therapy can help her develop the confidence to confront the people in her life whom she feels are treating her unfairly and to confront her own inability to state her needs. Career counseling is also useful to help her to examine her other options— and in most cases, there are other options. It may not happen overnight, but most people who want to make a job change and are willing to devote enough time and energy to the endeavor will eventually be able to do so.

When I refer patients to therapy or counseling, they often fear that they can't afford it. Most of the time, this isn't true. Many insurance companies will pay for part or even all of the cost of a licensed or state-certified therapist. In addition, there are many nonprofit mental health centers where patients are charged on a sliding scale based on their ability to pay. Although career counseling is not covered by medical insurance, nonprofit organizations such as the YWCA or the adult education department of your local college often offer counseling at reasonable fees. Sometimes, even employment agencies have resident career counselors who may also be able to place you in a job. With support from outside counseling, many of these "stuck" women realize that they do have the power to make positive changes in their lives.

Despite the sex role stereotyping, low pay, and all the other inequalities many women face in the workplace, women who work outside the home are generally healthier than homemakers. As a rule, they have fewer chronic illnesses, lower blood serum cholesterol levels, better HDL/LDL ratios, and a sense of being in better health. In short, multiple roles may be exhausting, but they can also be exhilarating, as well as offer emotional satisfaction and camaraderie that women who work in the solitary confinement of their own home may not feel.

Although many women derive a great deal of personal satisfaction from their jobs, they too may feel work-related stress, not only from what's going on in the office but from what they're "neglecting" at home. Often, women feel torn between their careers and their families. I know from my own experience that as soon as something goes wrong at home—a child comes home with a poor report card or gets sick at school—a woman's first thought is, "If I weren't working, this never would have happened." Men just aren't wired to think that way, but women almost always do and I know from firsthand experience that it can be very stressful.

I think any woman with small children is going to feel pulled between work and home, but there are ways of alleviating the guilt. First and foremost, you have to accept the fact that your job is not responsible for every calamity— minor or otherwise—that occurs at home or to your children. You must also accept another fact: Even women who stay at home with their children have kids who come home from school with black eyes, get occasional bad grades, or have other problems.

If a husband is not supportive of a wife's outside employment, it can be very upsetting for a woman, not only causing a serious strain on the marriage but actually imperiling her health. Even in a supportive relationship, a woman often feels torn between her work responsibility and her family, but in an unsupportive, difficult relationship, the pressure may become too overwhelming. These women in particular are at great risk of stress-related health problems and should seek marriage counseling, preferably with their husbands.

If a husband is verbally supportive but not much help around the house, it's important for you to communicate your need for extra help. Women are especially bad at doing this. They don't like to ask for help. And often, even if their husbands are willing to assume new responsibilities at home, they are reluctant to let them help on the grounds that they don't do a good enough job. But the question is, "Does it really matter if there are wrinkles on the bedspread, or whether or not Jason's shirt is the wrong shade of blue for his pants?" I don't think it really does. If by slightly lowering your standards you can find a few extra minutes a day to indulge in a bubble bath or read the newspaper, you are doing something positive for your body and your soul.

Chapter 13

A LETHAL
DOSE OF STRESS

STRESS is a double-edged sword. Not only is stress itself harmful to the body but the stressed-out woman often turns to unhealthy habits to help her cope. When she's keyed up after a long day at the office, she pours herself a stiff drink to relax. When she's nervous, she reaches for a cigarette. She may even seek relief by using cocaine or other illegal drugs. These "quick fixes," however, are not long-term solutions. In fact, ultimately they always aggravate the problem. Being dependent on alcohol, cigarettes, or any chemical substance is not only very stressful but can actually be lethal.

ALCOHOL

In our society, alcohol is such a commonly used drug that we often forget it is a drug. Alcohol (chemically known as ethanol) is an extremely potent drug that works by depressing the central nervous system. One or two drinks can make you feel relaxed and can enhance your sense of well-being. In social situations, alcohol can make you feel less inhibited and more outgoing. An occasional drink or two is not a problem for most people. In excess, however, alcohol can be very dangerous, especially for women. Women's bodies do not handle alcohol in exactly the same way as do men's. Women do not produce as much of a particular enzyme—alcohol dehydrogenase—needed to break down the alcohol molecule. Therefore, when we drink alcoholic beverages, we not only feel the effects of alcohol faster than men but it circulates longer throughout our body, making us susceptible to alcohol-related medical problems.

At 7 calories per milligram, alcohol is very fattening. A 3.5-ounce glass of wine is 100 calories. A mixed drink such as rum and coke weighs in at more than 300 calories. If you are a regular drinker, you may be consuming hundreds of extra calories daily, increasing your risk of obesity. Alcohol also raises blood triglyceride levels, a particularly important CAD risk factor for women. Even two drinks the night before a blood lipid profile may temporarily cause triglycerides to triple! If you consume alcohol every day, your triglycerides will be higher than if you don't. In fact, next to diabetes, excessive alcohol intake is the leading cause of hyperlipidemia. There have been some studies that show that one or two drinks a day increase HDL in some sedentary men and premenopausal women. However, I don't feel that the benefits of alcohol outweigh the drawbacks for women, especially since alcohol elevates triglycerides.

Alcohol also takes a steep toll on the cardiovascular system. Studies show that three or four drinks a day will cause a significant rise in blood pressure. In extremely high quantities, alcohol is also a poison that can actually kill heart cells. People who routinely consume extremely high levels of alcohol over a long period of time run the risk of cardiomyopathy, direct injury to heart tissue that can result in death. Fortunately, most of the damage reverses once the person stops drinking.

According to the National Center for Health Statistics, about 2.7 million women in the United States are alcohol-dependent, that is, they would experience actual withdrawal symptoms if they stopped drinking. These women are alcoholics. Another 1.8 million women are alcohol abusers, meaning they have an unhealthy relationship with alcohol. For example, a woman who drinks herself into a stupor every Saturday night but abstains all other times may not be alcohol-dependent, but she is certainly an abuser. Although frequency of drinking and quantity of alcohol consumed is one way of defining abuse, it is not the only way.

In *Now You Know*, Kitty Dukakis's revealing book about her chemical dependency, she confessed that during her husband's presidential campaign she would typically end her grueling day with one or two shots of vodka. From the minute she got up in the morning to her last campaign appearance, Mrs. Dukakis said that she looked forward to those drinks. Although the alcohol consumed at that time did not make her drunk, her reasons for drinking and her psychological dependency on alcohol constituted abuse. Eventually, after the campaign, when her drinking became much heavier, Mrs. Dukakis's family insisted that she receive treatment for her chemical dependency.

It was extremely courageous of Mrs. Dukakis to write so openly about her problems with alcohol. Women who are alcohol-dependent or abusers are typically so ashamed of their problem—or so unwilling to admit that they even have one—that they rarely step forward for help. In fact, family members often share in the disease and help these women hide and maintain their chemical dependency; this behavior is known as codependency. The woman and her family often do such a good job of denying and disguising the problem that her doctor is typically the last to know about it. Frankly, some physicians may also be blind to the problem, especially if the alcohol abuser is a middle-class or affluent woman who does not conform to the stereotype of the female drunk who lives at bars and collapses on the street.

Despite the negative stereotypes, in recent years it has become more accept-able for women to drink in public. As women have entered the work force, they have also entered the world of business lunches, conventions, and cock-tail parties. Therefore, many people assume that alcohol dependency and abuse must be on the rise among women. Many substance abuse experts, however, say that it is not true.

Although we may see more women drinking and hear more about women's drinking problems, alcohol abuse by women is nothing new. In fact, experts say that women's drinking patterns have not changed radically from the days when genteel women would become hooked on patent medicines that were primarily alcohol. Like the women alcohol abusers today, these women drank in the solitude of their homes. Unlike the male alcohol abuser who, at least some of the time, characteristically drinks in company, the female alcohol abuser usually drinks solo.

In general, women with drinking problems tend to be older than their male counterparts and drink less often than men, but they consume more alcohol during each binge. In my practice I have found that the isolated woman is particularly vulnerable to alcohol abuse, and on several occasions I have talked with these women about unhealthy drinking patterns. If I suspect that a patient has a problem with alcohol, I usually refer her to a physician who is a specialist in treating chemical dependency. Self-help groups such as Alco-holics Anonymous or Al Anon for family members can also be extremely beneficial.

What is a safe level of alcohol for women? If you are chemically dependent, no level of alcohol is safe. For most women, however, an occasional drink is not harmful as long as life does not revolve around it.

COCAINE

Taking cocaine is not chic—it's suicidal. Of the many drugs on which we can become dependent, cocaine is by far the most dangerous for the female heart. Over the past decade, cocaine has become the drug of choice for upper-income, recreational drug users, but cheaper forms such as crack have also made it a popular street drug. In its various forms, cocaine can be snorted, smoked—as in crack—or injected into the bloodstream. Cocaine produces a "high" that makes the user feel euphoric, but at great expense to the cardio-vascular system.

There is more than one way that cocaine can affect the heart: It can cause coronary artery spasm, reducing the flow of oxygen to the heart, which can result in a heart attack. Cocaine can also trigger an arrhythmia, which in some cases can be lethal. There is no safe level of cocaine: Any dose can be fatal, especially if the user has a cardiac condition that makes her prone to arrhythmia, such as mitral valve prolapse. If taken during pregnancy, cocaine greatly increases the odds that the baby will be born with a serious congenital heart defect. Sadly, an estimated 10 percent of all pregnant women in the United States use cocaine, and this figure may be as high as 50 percent in some urban areas. Our inability to prevent the spread of this drug is a tragedy that is going to haunt us for decades to come.

SMOKING

About 27 percent of all women smoke, and although that number reflects a decline of 6 percent since 1965, it is still alarmingly high. For one thing, women are not quitting at the same rate as men (who showed a 20 percent decline during the same period). For another, a million teenagers take up smoking every year, many of them female. In fact, 18.1 percent of all female high school seniors smoke as compared to 17.4 percent of the males. We hear from our own children that young college women are now joining their male classmates in chewing as well as smoking tobacco.

Most young women start to smoke because they think it's sophisticated or grown up. Studies show, however, that once hooked, women turn to cigarettes for different reasons, often to help them cope with frustration and anger. Despite the well-publicized health risks, many women also use smoking as a tool to stay thin. When they feel the urge to eat, they reach for a cigarette.

As the surgeon general's warning on every cigarette package clearly states, smoking can be dangerous to your health. With every puff that you take, you are inhaling a hot stream of chemicals—including tar and carbon monoxide—that can inflict severe damage on your throat, lungs, and even your arteries. In fact, smokers can develop a very specific type of arteriosclerotic lesion. Women who smoke also run a greater risk of developing lung cancer, which recently has surpassed breast cancer as the leading cancer killer of women.

Tobacco also contains nicotine, a potent and potentially addictive chemical that affects the brain and central nervous system, both exciting the body and relaxing it at the same time. When you inhale cigarette smoke, your heartbeat increases, your blood vessels constrict, and your peripheral circulation slows down. The brain releases alpha waves, associated with a relaxed state, and also triggers the release of endorphins, chemicals that provide a feeling of well-being. Although nicotine may make you feel good, it is not good for you. In fact, studies suggest that it promotes blood clots, which could explain why smokers have a higher rate of stroke than nonsmokers. Smokers are also at greater risk of high blood pressure, heart attack, emphysema, and many respiratory disorders. Women who smoke become menopausal earlier than normal, further increasing their risk of CAD.

Smoking also has a bad effect on blood lipids. According to a recent study, compared to nonsmokers, smokers on average have cholesterol levels that are 3 percent higher, triglyceride levels that are 9 percent higher, LDLs ("bad" cholesterol) that are 12 percent higher, and HDLs ("good" cholesterol) that are 6 percent lower.

Obviously, if you smoke you should try to stop. I realize that it is easier said than done. Many smokers experience severe withdrawal symptoms when they quit, including headaches, change in appetite, insomnia, constipation, increased anxiety, and even tremors. For some people, these symptoms disappear within a week or so, but for others they linger for weeks or even months.

Women have an especially difficult time when they try to kick the habit, as demonstrated by their poorer success rates in smoking cessation programs. Researchers are not sure whether biological differences actually make it more difficult for women to quit smoking, or whether other factors are to blame. For example, many women are afraid that if they stop smoking they will gain weight. Many smokers do experience a temporary slowdown in their metabolism when they quit, which often leads to weight gain, but eventually their bodies adjust to the change. If weight gain is an issue, women should receive nutritional counseling from a registered dietitian while they are attempting to quit smoking.

In addition, if a woman has become accustomed to using cigarettes as a means of coping with her stress and frustration, she must find other outlets for her pent-up emotions before she can successfully stop. Before she begins a smoking cessation program, she must deal with the feelings that are driving her to light up. Often, counseling can be useful to help these women develop coping skills that will decrease their dependence on cigarettes.

Because it is often so difficult to stop smoking, I frequently refer patients to smoking cessation programs, such as those run by the local chapters of the American Lung Association or Smokenders. Although quitting is difficult, it is not impossible. According to the American Lung Association, more than 40 million Americans have already quit, and thus dramatically reduced their risk of premature death.

RESOURCES: For information on treating addictions and how to find support groups, see pages 233 to 234.

VI

WHEN THINGS
GO WRONG

❧

Chapter 14

A GUIDE TO
TESTS AND NUMBERS

THERE are two kinds of women with heart disease: those who know it and those who don't. For every woman who comes to me complaining of telltale signs such as chest pains or breathlessness, there is another whose body is being silently ravaged by CAD. Neither she nor her doctor may realize what is happening until the damage has been done. The fact that she has no symptoms is no guarantee that she doesn't have heart disease or that she has not had a heart attack. Therefore, it is absolutely critical that doctors consider the possibility that even a symptomless woman might have heart disease, especially if she is postmenopausal or has other risk factors.

If a patient complains of symptoms such as chest pain, heart palpitations, or dizziness, or if during a careful examination a doctor suspects that a patient may have CAD, she will refer her for further testing.

There have been some dazzling technological breakthroughs in the past decade or so that aid us immeasurably in determining the extent of heart disease, but as you will see, tests results are only as good as the person who is interpreting them. Therefore, every woman needs to be monitored by a doctor who can evaluate those test results in the context of her lifestyle and medical history.

This chapter contains information on state-of-the-art diagnostic tools that doctors use to detect heart disease, when those tests are necessary, and what the results really mean. Although technology can enhance our diagnostic skills, I believe there is no substitute for good, old-fashioned, hands-on medicine. Diagnosing heart disease takes a great deal more than a battery of tests. A good rapport with the patient is essential. A caring doctor armed with only a stethoscope, who actually talks and listens to her patients, may know more about her patient's health than one who rushes through the examination, relying solely on fancy equipment to make a diagnosis.

If your doctor suspects that you may have had a heart attack within the past few days, she will send a sample of your blood to a laboratory to be analyzed for certain key substances called myocardial enzymes that are found in the blood when part of the heart muscle dies.

In some cases, your doctor may order additional tests to assess chest pain and to decide whether it is, in fact, due to a heart attack. For example, if she suspects that your chest pain may actually be related to a digestive problem such as an ulcer or a hiatal hernia, she may order a gastrointestinal (GI) series or X ray of the stomach and esophagus to confirm her diagnosis.

ELECTROCARDIOGRAM (EKG)

1. *What is it?* This painless, noninvasive test is performed at rest. A jellylike substance is rubbed on the chest, arms, and legs. Electrodes, attached either with adhesive or by rubber straps, are placed over these areas. Twelve wires attached to the electrodes feed into the electrocardiographic machine and a record of the heart's electrical activity is recorded.

2. *What does it mean?* The lines or waves that result appear in a definite pattern that are identified by letters *P-QRS-T* (see diagram on page 153). The *P* wave measures electrical activity in the atria. Waves *QRS* and *T* measure electrical activity in the ventricles. (For some unknown reason, after puberty the length of the *Q-T* interval in women is slightly longer than that of men at the same heart rates.) The EKG is done on special calibrated or graph paper so that exact measurements can be made. The physician uses a special caliper to make her measurements. From the EKG, the doctor can assess whether the rhythm is regular, originating from the proper place, and whether or not there is any sign of injury to the heart muscle or to its covering, the pericardium. The doctor can also detect the possibility of enlargement of one or more chambers of the heart. She can also see evidence of old scarring.

The EKG cannot always diagnose damage to the heart: In fact, it will be normal for about 50 percent of all patients who complain of angina, although they may have CAD.

The EKG reflects the heart's activity for as long as the leads are attached to the patient. It cannot predict future problems. For the half hour or so that we monitor the patient in the office, everything may be working perfectly. But there's no guarantee that once the EKG leads are removed and the patient has gone home she will not suddenly experience a period of silent ischemia—that is, suffer a temporary reduction in oxygen to her heart cells because of spasm of her coronary arteries. She may also develop a serious arrhythmia. So although the EKG is a useful diagnostic tool, it alone cannot completely reassure the patient or her doctor. If a patient has a normal EKG and no

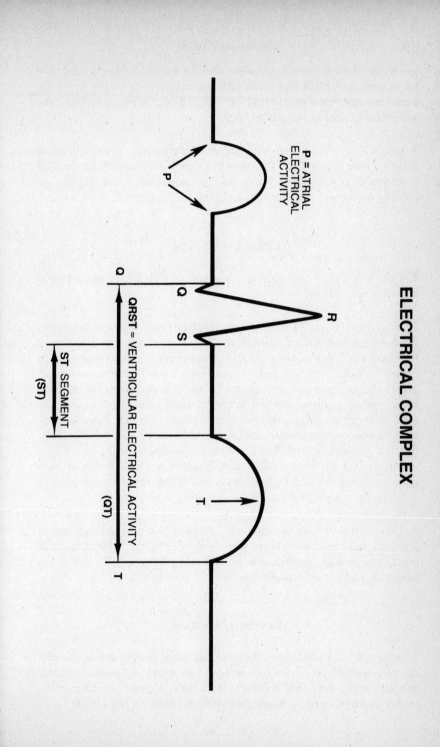

ELECTRICAL COMPLEX

P = ATRIAL
ELECTRICAL
ACTIVITY

QRST = VENTRICULAR ELECTRICAL ACTIVITY

ST SEGMENT
(ST)

(QT)

P

Q

R

S

T

symptoms, she will probably not require further testing. If, however, a patient has an abnormal EKG, symptoms such as chest pains, or for any reason the doctor suspects that a patient may have CAD or another heart problem, she will probably recommend further tests.

3. *Who is it for?* Any woman who complains of chest pain, heart palpitations or shows other signs of CAD should be given an EKG. Since 35 percent of all heart attacks in women are "silent" and go undetected, I routinely give an EKG to any woman over forty as part of her annual physical.

HOLTER MONITOR

1. *What is it?* The Holter monitor is a small, portable EKG that the patient actually wears at home.

2. *What does it mean?* This device monitors the heart's rhythm and can also show changes that may indicate "silent ischemia" or a temporary reduction of the blood supply to the heart muscle because of coronary artery spasm. Some of these episodes occur in response to everyday stresses. Therefore, patients are asked to keep a log of their activities for 24 hours. By comparing the log to the Holter recordings, the doctor can determine which, if any, specific activities seem to trigger problems, and conversely, whether or not the patient's symptoms are connected to unusual cardiac events. Because it uses only two leads, this test provides less information than the complete EKG. But it does something that the office EKG cannot: It detects any arrhythmias or silent ischemic attacks that may typically occur during the course of a day, but may not show up in an hour at rest on the examining table.

3. *Who is it for?* A doctor prescribes a Holter if a patient complains of dizziness, heart palpitations, chest pain, fainting episodes, or if the EKG itself reveals one or more premature beats, indicating the possibility that an arrhythmia might or did actually develop from time to time.

ECHOCARDIOGRAM

1. *What is it?* An EKG shows the heart's electrical activity, but an echocardiogram actually provides a picture of the structure of the heart. In this painless, noninvasive test, a transducer or wand is passed over the chest, producing and picking up sound waves reflected from the heart itself.

2. *What does it mean?* The resulting pattern produces a three-dimensional picture of the heart on a screen. You may already be familiar with this technology in another context: During pregnancy, many women are routinely given sonograms, which also use sound waves to create a picture of the fetus. In the case of an echocardiogram, the picture produced by the sound waves can tell us a great deal about the anatomy and functioning of the heart. An echocardiogram will show the size of the chambers and image any portion of the heart that does not contract properly. When combined with a Doppler to measure the amount and direction of blood flow, it can also trace the flow of blood through the nooks and crannies of the heart to detect any valve problems such as holes in the septa between the chambers (which cause shunting of blood in the wrong direction). Unfortunately, an echocardiogram is not useful in determining whether or not the coronary arteries are diseased or narrowed. It can only find the scars of old injury, and even that, only sometimes.

If the echocardiogram shows signs of ventricular enlargement, or poor function that suggests the patient may have already had a heart attack, I advise the patient to have an exercise stress test.

3. *Who is it for?* I would prescribe an echocardiogram for any patient with unexplained and possible cardiac symptoms, for those with an abnormal EKG to check for damaged portions of the heart muscle, or in any situation where more information is needed on the anatomy of the heart. For example, if a patient has hypertension, I might order an echocardiogram to see if the heart has become enlarged.

EXERCISE STRESS TEST

1. *What is it?* This test combines rigorous exercise—either walking on a treadmill or riding a stationary bicycle—with an EKG. The purpose is to determine whether or not the heart is getting enough oxygen during times of activity, and to detect any possible life-threatening arrhythmias that may develop during periods of emotional or physical stress. As in the standard resting EKG, 12 leads are placed on the patient's body: on all four extremities and across the chest. Then, while monitored by a trained physician, she is told to begin exercising, slowly at first, until she reaches a predetermined target heart rate based on her age and physical condition. The heart rate is measured by monitoring the patient's pulse. Her blood pressure is also monitored throughout the test by the same physician.

2. *What does it mean?* If the patient experiences any untoward symptoms such as intolerable fatigue or chest pain during exercise, if she develops a serious arrhythmia, or if her *S-T* segment (part of the pattern of each electrical complex the heart generates) becomes depressed, it might mean that the patient is suffering from a lack of oxygen, due to a narrowing of a coronary artery. Usually, the stress test will not detect a problem unless one or more coronary arteries are at least 50 percent blocked, so this test is not useful in diagnosing early stages of CAD. Under the best of circumstances, the stress test will only identify 65 percent of all patients with CAD. In other words, in 35 percent of all cases, patients who actually have the disease will be given a clean bill of health.

About 10 percent of the time, the stress test will show CAD in people who don't have it, typically misdiagnosing "false positives" in women more than in men. The accuracy of the stress test depends on an accurate reading, which is why I always insist on seeing the raw data myself. For one thing, it is absolutely critical to consider factors such as the patient's sex, age, menopausal state, lipid profile, and symptoms when weighing the significance of a test result. It is also important to consider exactly at what point during the test an abnormality occurred. For example, if someone developed an abnormal heartbeat early in the test after a low level of exertion, I would be very concerned. I would be even more concerned if that person's blood pressure suddenly dropped, if her pulse weakened, or if she became faint or light-headed. In these situations, the test should be discontinued and the results should be taken very seriously. If just a little exercise causes these types of problems, this person may be at serious risk of a heart attack.

Although the risks are minimal, there have been cases of sudden death during stress tests due to the unexpected onset of a lethal arrhythmia. In addition, for patients with certain problems—specifically those with severe aortic stenosis, characterized by extreme narrowing of the aortic valve, or certain types of arrhythmias—the test can be fatal. I would hope that patients with these conditions do not take a stress test, but at times these problems may go undiagnosed. Therefore, the stress test should only be performed by a physician who is prepared to resuscitate a patient in the unlikely event that it is necessary.

3. *Who is it for?* I recommend this test for any patient with an abnormal EKG or angina. A modified stress test is usually given to patients after a heart attack before they are discharged from the hospital. I also recommend an exercise stress test to any woman over forty who is embarking on an exercise program and has one or more risk factors for CAD. If more information is needed after the standard exercise stress test, I order it repeated with the addition of a thallium tracer.

THALLIUM EXERCISE STRESS TEST

1. What is it? This procedure uses a radioactive substance to trace the flow of blood through the heart. Similar to the exercise stress test, a patient exercises up to her predetermined heart rate. Then a tiny amount of thallium, a radioactive material, is injected into a vein. The patient lies down on the examining table as a special camera monitors the distribution of thallium as it is taken up from the blood by the myocardial, or heart, cells.

2. What does it mean? If a portion of the heart does not receive thallium, it's safe to assume that the area is being denied blood. The imaging of the radioactivity of the heart is then repeated some hours later while the patient is at rest. In some cases, the later test done at rest is normal, showing that the heart is only temporarily being denied blood during times of maximum work. If the second test is abnormal too, it means that part of the heart (the part that shows no radioactivity) may have been permanently damaged, probably due to a heart attack.

Depending on the problem, medication may be prescribed to improve the flow of blood through the heart, or other treatments may be considered. The thallium stress test diagnoses CAD with 90 percent accuracy in both men and women, so although it's not perfect, it's a lot better than the regular exercise stress test. However, in rare cases, female contours and breast tissue can sometimes interfere with the physician's ability to get a clear picture.

3. Who is it for? If the standard exercise stress test is inconclusive, or if I strongly suspect that a patient has CAD, I might refer them for the thallium stress test. We do not perform this test routinely. For one thing, the thallium test is much more expensive than the regular stress test, and for another, it takes a lot longer to perform. Frankly, I feel that diagnostic tests themselves can be stressful, and I don't like to subject my patients to them unless they are absolutely necessary. If I need more information after the thallium test, I refer patients for catheterization.

CARDIAC CATHETERIZATION AND ANGIOGRAPHY

1. What is it? In cardiac catheterization, a plastic tube is passed through a blood vessel in the arm or thigh into the heart. It is performed in a hospital under local anesthesia and is usually painless. In coronary angiography, a dye is injected into the catheter and an X ray follows the dye as it flows through the coronary arteries throughout the heart. The patient may feel a momentary rush of heat or discomfort when the dye is injected.

2. *What does it mean?* Up until now, all of the diagnostic tests we have discussed are useful to detect evidence of CAD. But only cardiac catheterization can conclusively show whether or not the coronary arteries are diseased, which vessels are affected, where the blockage is located, and by how much the artery is narrowed. We can also see whether the flow of blood has been detoured to collateral blood vessels—blood vessels that develop when heart muscle is chronically deprived of oxygen. From all of this information, we can determine the patient's likelihood of having a serious heart attack.

Despite other diagnostic innovations, coronary angiography is still the gold standard when it comes to diagnosing CAD. It is not only highly accurate but provides specific information that cannot be obtained through any other means. Unfortunately, there is a price to pay for this information: It is riskier than other nonsurgical procedures. In fact, 1 out of 500 patients will have a heart attack, stroke, or other serious complication due to catheterization. In my opinion, this procedure should not be performed unless it is absolutely necessary.

3. *Who is it for?* Candidates for bypass surgery or angioplasty must be catheterized to evaluate the likely success of either procedure. I also recommend catheterization to patients who show a sudden change for the worse. For example, if a patient who had previously been controlling her angina with medication suddenly complains of more frequent and painful chest pains, I would order a catheterization to see exactly what was going on. She may need different medication, or she might require balloon angioplasty or even bypass surgery.

ON THE HORIZON

Although they are not used routinely now, there are some interesting technological developments that may one day aid in the diagnosis of CAD. A case in point is magnetic resonance imaging, or MRI, which is now used to detect brain tumors, among other things. By using powerful magnets to look inside the body, MRI provides a wonderful picture of the heart, and in some medical facilities it is even used to help identify damage after a heart attack. However, its usefulness for diagnosing CAD is limited, because unless there is calcium in the coronary artery wall, it will not reveal whether the artery is narrowed.

Positron emission topography (PET) scan is another example of state-of-the-art technology that may prove to be a useful tool in diagnosing CAD. PET scan provides information about cardiac metabolism: It shows how the heart uses food to get energy. Although this information is interesting, as of yet there is no application for the diagnosis of heart disease—we simply don't know how to use it.

Perhaps one day there will be a simple, noninvasive, diagnostic test that will detect CAD with 100 percent accuracy. As things stand now, however, there is no substitute for cardiac catheterization.

Chapter 15

HAVING A
HEART ATTACK

THIS chapter may be the most important one in the book because it contains information that could save your life. I will describe exactly what a heart attack is, what to do if you think that you're having one, the different treatment options that are available, and how you and your physician can help bring about your full recovery. But before I give you this vital information, I want to tell you about one of my patients, Mary Logan, so that you don't make the same mistake that she did.

Mary Logan, age fifty-five, woke up one winter morning feeling achy, nauseated, and more exhausted than when she went to sleep. Mary assumed that she must have caught a touch of flu from her husband, John, who was back at work for the first day after two weeks in bed. Nevertheless, she had planned on cleaning out the upstairs bedroom closets that day in anticipation of a week-long visit by her grandchildren, and so she dragged herself out of bed, got dressed, and immediately got to work. By midmorning she felt a sense of pressure in the middle of her chest that traveled across her chest down her left arm. This time, Mary assumed that she must have lifted something the wrong way and that she had strained a muscle. Within a few minutes, the pressure changed to pain, and Mary slumped into her bedroom chair, waiting to feel better.

Although Mary could easily have reached for the telephone without getting up, she did not call anyone for help. John was in business meetings all day and she did not want to disturb him. Her daughter, Ruth, who lived nearby, was busy with her new baby and Mary did not want to disturb her. And why should she bother her doctor when she knew that all he would probably do was tell her to get more rest? So Mary sat in her chair for an hour until her daughter finally called her. Upon hearing her mother's weakened voice, Ruth rushed over to the house to check on her. She was shocked by what she saw: Her mother's face was ashen, her forehead and upper lip were beaded with sweat, and her expression was anxious.

Ruth immediately took her mother to the nearest emergency room. It's a good thing that she did—Mary was having a heart attack. Some of the cells in her heart muscle were dying due to lack of oxygen. An EKG revealed that Mary's heartbeat was dangerously irregular. Without immediate care, her heart could have developed a lethal arrhythmia that could have killed her. Fortunately, prompt medical intervention saved Mary's life. If her daughter had not taken her to the hospital, I believe Mary would have been 1 of 247,000 women who die of heart attack each year, many within the first hour or so of the attack.

Anyone reading this story may think that it is ridiculous. How can anyone mistake anything as serious as a heart attack for the flu or even muscle strain? But based on decades of experience, I'm more surprised by the patient who steps forward early in the game and says, "I'm having a heart attack. Help me!" When it comes to heart attacks, there is a great deal of denial on the part of all patients in general, and women patients in particular. Studies show that the average heart attack victim waits between two and five hours to call her doctor. (Interestingly enough, there is no relationship between the severity of the attack and the delay time.) Women are more likely than men not to call the doctor at all. In fact, more than one third of all heart attacks in women go unnoticed or unreported by their victims.

Some women may be too frightened to even acknowledge the possibility that they are having a heart. It's also true that for many women a heart attack may seem so unlikely that they are completely unaware of the warning signs. Therefore, I'm now going to discuss how you can tell when you're having a heart attack. At the first sign of a problem, call your physician or get to the nearest emergency room. Remember that even if you are mistaken and it turns out to be nothing more than indigestion or some other minor problem, it's better to be overly cautious than to be dead wrong.

AM I HAVING A HEART ATTACK?

You could be having a heart attack if you are experiencing any of the following symptoms:

1. Intense pressure or crushing pain in your chest. The sensation may travel down your arms, into your neck, or may even begin in the back. It will last for two minutes or more. Patients often describe the sensation as feeling "as if an elephant is sitting on my chest." If you have angina, you may worry that you won't be able to distinguish between a temporary ischemic attack and the real thing. But believe me, in most cases, you will. Often, the pain of a heart attack is much more severe, lasts for a

longer period of time, and will not go away if you take oral nitro-glycerine. Although rest often helps reduce or stop the pain of angina, it offers little comfort against the bone-crushing pain of a full-blown heart attack. In fact, you may be in such discomfort that it is literally impossible to sit still. Patients often pace frantically, often in such agony that they don't know what to do with themselves. One famous cardiologist described finding one of his patients hanging his arms from a doorjamb in an effort to relieve the pain he was experiencing.

2. A feeling of faintness or light-headedness.
3. A sensation of difficulty in breathing or shortness of breath.
4. A feeling of severe, intense indigestion that doesn't go away after taking an antacid or burping.
5. A feeling of impending doom, that something terrible is happening, that death is imminent. Some patients claim to experience this.

Just because you're experiencing one or more of these symptoms doesn't necessarily mean that you are having a heart attack. There are times when chest pain may indeed be just indigestion or even the first warning of an ulcer. A sharp pain in the back can mean a muscle or bone injury. I know that it may be embarrassing for a patient to rush to the emergency room only to be told by some intern to take two antacids and call the doctor in the morning. But believe me, for every patient who summons me out of bed in the middle of the night for a false alarm, there are others who are truly in crises. And I would prefer that my patients call me the first minute they even suspect that they're having a heart attack rather than suffer an attack without attention.

Patients often ask me if there are any early clues that could be a precursor of an impending heart attack. Unfortunately, often there aren't any. In many cases, a heart attack seems to strike out of nowhere. An active, vigorous person suddenly begins to feel chest pains, and before she knows it she's in the coronary care unit. Others do have warning signs, but they're so subtle that they often go unrecognized. For instance, many of my patients tell me that for a month or two leading up to their heart attacks they felt simply drained and exhausted. I can't say for sure why this would be, except perhaps that they were already experiencing a lack of oxygen due to an obstruction of the coronary arteries, which might cause excessive fatigue.

In addition, heart attacks often occur after periods of extreme physical or emotional stress. If you are unusually tired for two or more weeks, and know that you are at risk for a heart attack, it might be a good idea to see your doctor just to make sure you're okay. Only 15 percent of all heart attacks happen during times of extreme exertion, for example, the weekend athlete collapsing on the tennis court or the high-powered attorney keeling over during a tense

negotiation. In most other cases, the heart attack strikes during times of rest, typically on vacation or even right after getting up in the morning. In fact, early morning is an extremely vulnerable time for the heart due to bodily rhythms stimulating hormonal secretions that promote blood clots. A blood clot can lodge in a coronary artery, blocking the blood flow to the heart. So if you get out of bed experiencing any symptoms that may be related to a heart attack, don't wait—call your doctor and get to an emergency room.

Having warned you about the symptoms of heart attack, and the importance of not ignoring them, I have to tell you that in some cases there will be no symptoms. You might have a heart attack without feeling any pain at all—in fact, you may not even know if you've had one. A small portion of heart muscle could have died. The heart could have adjusted to the loss, and you would be none the wiser.

Anywhere between 25 percent and 40 percent of all myocardial infarctions may be silent heart attacks that are revealed sometime later on a routine EKG. The silent heart attack could be a prelude to a bigger and more damaging one, or it could be a solitary event that will never happen again. Although we don't know why some heart attacks are painless, we suspect that women get silent heart attacks more often than men simply because women are less likely to report a heart attack to their doctors.

I personally wonder whether in some cases women deny or ignore symptoms. But silent heart attacks are real heart attacks. They can be every bit as damaging as heart attacks that scream to be noticed. We may not know when they're happening, but we can do a lot to prevent them. Thus, it is critical for people who are at risk of developing CAD to be closely monitored by their physicians, and their risk factors should be carefully managed.

What to Do If You Think You're Having a Heart Attack

When any medical emergency strikes, including a heart attack, most people are understandably paralyzed with fear. Precious minutes can be lost fumbling for the doctor's phone number, looking up the name of the ambulance service, or checking the location of the nearest hospital. Therefore, it is advisable to work out an emergency plan with your doctor ahead of time. By the way, remember that when you choose a doctor you are also indirectly choosing the hospital where you will be treated in times of emergency. Typically, doctors are affiliated with one or more hospitals where they can admit patients. As part of your emergency plan, you should ask your doctor about the hospital in which she works. If you are at risk for heart disease, I suggest that you find a doctor who is affiliated with a hospital that has a state-of-the-art coronary care unit.

Remember to inform other family members in your household or a trustworthy neighbor about any emergency plan you may devise with your doctor. Keep important phone numbers—your doctor's, the local ambulance service, your spouse's work number—and directions to the hospital posted near the telephone. Remember that in some cases you may be unconscious or too ill to give instructions. You and your doctor should discuss ahead of time what you should do and where you should go in case of a medical emergency. Your doctor will probably tell you to call her office or her answering service as soon as you experience any symptoms that remotely resemble a heart attack, especially if you are a high-risk patient. Make sure that you tell the nurse or operator that it is not a routine call: Say specifically, "I think I am having a heart attack. I need to talk to the doctor." In an ideal world, your doctor will get back to you immediately and probably tell you to meet her in the emergency room of the hospital in which she is affiliated. Your doctor will then call ahead so that the emergency room staff is prepared for your arrival.

But your doctor may be tending to another emergency or may be otherwise unavailable. In this case, go directly to the emergency room. By the way, never drive yourself—there's a risk of fainting or blacking out behind the wheel. Get a friend or relative to take you, preferably someone who can stay with you until you have received treatment. When you arrive at the emergency room, once again make sure that you or your companion clearly states to the triage nurse—the person who decides who gets treated first—that you are having a heart attack. Don't be vague or uncertain: Don't say "I think I'm having a heart attack." Say "I am having a heart attack. I need to see a doctor right now." Emergency rooms are very busy places, and if you want immediate attention you had better present yourself as a true emergency.

IN THE AMBULANCE AND AT THE HOSPITAL

I have said repeatedly that it is essential to notify your doctor and get to the hospital as early as possible if you even suspect that you're having a heart attack. During a heart attack, medically known as a myocardial infarction, portions of heart muscle are dying due to a lack of oxygen. As you know by now, the coronary arteries feed blood to the heart. If the arteries become extremely narrowed, or if a blood clot or piece of plaque lodges inside of an artery, the blood supply to portions of the heart muscle will be cut off.

Arteriosclerosis—clogging of the arteries with lipid deposits—is a leading cause of heart attack, but not the only cause. In fact, in 6 percent of all heart attacks, and 24 percent of all heart attacks in patients under thirty-five, there is no evidence of CAD. What caused the heart attack? Sometimes a congenital problem, such as aortic stenosis, or narrowing of the aorta, may reduce the blood flow to the heart. A blow to the chest can trigger a heart attack. In other cases, often involving women, a coronary artery may go into spasm, choking off the blood flow to part of the heart.

Cocaine can cause the coronary arteries to go into spasm, thus cutting off the heart's oxygen supply. Prolonged periods of extreme stress can also cause the coronary arteries to constrict or narrow, reducing the oxygen flow. There are even diseases that can cause inflammation of the blood vessels, which can result in reduced blood flow. Whatever the cause of the heart attack, if the oxygen supply is not returned within four to six hours, the damage is irreversible. No matter what we do, those cells are dead forever. If everything is working well, other cells will eventually pick up the slack, taking over the jobs performed by the dead cells. But if the damage is too extensive, the remaining cells may not be able to do all the necessary work to keep the heart pumping.

Obviously, once a heart attack begins, it's critical to get the blood circulating throughout the heart as soon as possible to minimize the damage. If you take an ambulance to the hospital, you will probably be given oxygen immediately by the attendant to improve the oxygen content of whatever blood is circulating throughout the heart. You may also be given morphine, which not only helps relieve the pain but reduces the terrible anxiety that often accompanies a heart attack and can put an added strain on the heart. The attendant will also monitor your heartbeat with an EKG to detect any dangerous arrhythmias. If you are showing signs of a life-threatening arrhythmia, the attendant or physician may use a defibrillator to give the heart an electric shock to restore normal heart rhythm.

If you go directly to the hospital yourself, you will probably be taken to a special room for cardiac cases where the attending physician will examine you. He will also give you oxygen, administer painkiller if you need it, and take an EKG. In most cases, irregularities on the EKG will confirm that you are having a heart attack, or that you've recently had one. However, even if the EKG does not show any irregularities, the doctor may keep you for further testing. In some cases, the doctor may order special blood tests to determine if any heart muscle has died.

After a heart attack, the dying heart cells secrete special chemicals called enzymes that appear in the bloodstream hours after the attack. They peak at different times, but all disappear within three to four days. If the blood test is positive for these enzymes, it almost always means that you had a heart attack. If the physician feels that you may be in heart failure, that is, your heart is not pumping properly and fluid is pooling either in the lungs or in the rest of the body, he will give you a diuretic to rid your body of excess fluid.

If you get to the hospital within the first three hours after the inception of the heart attack, it may be possible to stop and even reverse the damage with reperfusion therapy: dissolving the clot that is blocking the flow of blood. A new class of drugs popularly known as "clot busters" may be given to help open up the affected artery. In some parts of the United States and Europe, these drugs are administered in the ambulance.

Clot busters are not for everyone. In the process of breaking up the clot in the coronary artery, they can cause severe bleeding in another part of the body. Therefore, they can be especially dangerous for people with a history of bleeding ulcers, blood in the stool, diverticulosis, heavy menstrual periods, or bleeding between periods. Thus, I believe that these drugs should only be administered by a physician in an emergency room who is aware of the patient's medical history. Keep in mind that a patient who is suffering a heart attack may be in no position to give an accurate account of her past health; therefore, it is especially critical that her regular physician be in touch with the emergency room staff.

The different types of clot-dissolving agents are either administered through an IV or injected directly into the coronary arteries via a catheter. Streptokinase and urokinase are enzymes that are commonly used to break up blood clots. If you get to the hospital within the first hour of the heart attack, it may be possible to use a relatively new drug called tissue plasminogen activator, or TPA, which helps stimulate the body to produce its own clot-dissolving agents. If you are given any of these clot busters, you must be catheterized within 18 to 24 hours to make sure the clot is gone.

In some cases, if you get to the hospital within that critical six-hour period, your cardiologist may decide to perform a balloon angioplasty to open the artery. A catheter with a deflated balloon on its tip is passed into the place where the coronary artery is narrowed. When the balloon is inflated, the plaque causing the obstruction is then flattened against the artery wall and the lumen is reopened. Balloon angioplasty should be performed only by highly skilled physicians who have a great deal of experience in this procedure.

If you arrive at the hospital early enough, and an aggressive surgical team is on hand, your physician may opt for emergency bypass surgery to restore oxygen to your heart. The surgeon takes a blood vessel from another part of the body and constructs a detour around the blocked section of coronary artery.

In reality, early intervention—the kind that minimizes the damage to the heart, and in some cases, reverses it—is usually impractical. Most patients wait at least two hours into a heart attack before calling the doctor. By the time they arrive at the hospital, they are probably no longer candidates for clot busters. In addition, although theoretically possible, other more "heroic" procedures may be impractical. In order to have bypass surgery or balloon angioplasty, a skilled, experienced surgical team must be on hand at a moment's notice. If you have a heart attack at 3 A.M., it is unlikely that the team will be there, unless your doctor is able to arrange for a surgeon to come to the hospital. (I have gotten many of my colleagues out of bed late at night to help one of my patients, and the quid pro quo is that I am willing to do the same thing for their patients! Talk to your doctor about this ahead of time.)

More likely than not, after you are examined by the emergency room physician you will spend the next 24 to 36 hours in the coronary care unit, or CCU. In the CCU, you will be closely monitored until your condition is stabilized—that is, until you are out of pain and show no signs of heart failure or dangerous arrhythmia, which is a leading cause of sudden death. A specially trained cardiac team will monitor your every breath; a bedside monitor will record your every heartbeat. A catheter may be inserted through a vein in your neck and threaded into your right ventricle to measure your blood pressure. Often, during times of acute stress, such as a heart attack, blood pressure may soar, increasing the work of the heart just at a time when the heart is already in overdrive. Therefore, it is critical to keep blood pressure within normal levels.

Sometimes a few reassuring words from the physician is all it takes to relax the patient and bring the blood pressure down. If that doesn't work, medication may be required. If your blood pressure is in the stratosphere, you may be given nitroprusside through an IV, which usually brings it right down. Some physicians may give beta blockers to slow down the heart, thus reducing its workload. Others prefer to use ACE inhibitors, drugs that help the heart contract and also improve the flow of blood to the kidneys. Sometimes a combination of different drugs is required.

You may also be given medication to control any arrhythmia, or a cardiotonic drug such as digitalis to help your heart beat more strongly. If you are feeling pain—a sign that cells are still dying or at risk of dying—you may be given nitroglycerine to relax the muscle tone of the arteries and veins, thus allowing the blood to flow more freely. It is important to remember that during times of acute crises such as a heart attack there is no one correct approach: It is very much a judgment call on the part of the physician, who must be on hand every minute to respond to the patient's needs.

In terms of pure human drama, there is no place in the hospital quite like the CCU. Every patient is in crisis—physically and emotionally. Since these special units first appeared on the scene in the 1960s, death from heart attack has dropped an astounding 25 percent! CCUs are generally the best-staffed part of the hospital. In some hospitals, there is one nurse for every patient. The nurses are specially trained to deal with cardiac crises. They are usually highly professional and extremely dedicated.

As wonderful as this care can be, there are some disadvantages to being so closely watched. Because every patient must be in full view of the nursing staff, the CCU resembles one large ward with each bed separated from the next by a mere curtain or a windowed partition. There is no privacy. The noise is incessant. It is very difficult to escape the constant turmoil that is going on around you. The patient in the next bed goes into cardiac arrest and suddenly a team of doctors and nurses descend upon his bed and try to revive him. Another is being wheeled out with a sheet over his face. Anxious relatives hover about. Every few hours, a nurse comes by to give you medication or to take another test. The lights are always on whether it is day or night. Getting a few hours of undisturbed sleep is nearly an impossibility.

Not surprisingly, many patients in the CCU become profoundly anxious. To begin with, after a heart attack you feel frightened and vulnerable. Your anxiety is compounded by the lack of sleep and the sight of other acutely ill patients. Many CCU patients are overcome by an overwhelming sense of terror. Some patients even begin to hallucinate. These emotions are called coronary care unit psychosis. At times of such crises, it is extremely important to be able to talk openly about your feelings with your physician. It's important to understand that your depression and anxiety are quite normal. I view it as a healthy sign when a patient shows the appropriate range of negative emotions in the CCU. She is acting normally in a very abnormal situation.

At the same time, the crisis atmosphere in the CCU can sometimes have a positive effect on a patient and her family. Like the jolt of electricity that gives order to a chaotic heartbeat, a visit to the CCU can often shock a family back into reality. Suddenly, the petty differences that kept family members apart no longer seem all that important. Estranged children rush to their parent's bedside. Siblings who have been out of touch for years show up to lend their support. Husbands and wives who may have been drifting apart suddenly rediscover each other. I don't mean to romanticize what it's like to be a patient in the CCU—believe me, given any choice in the matter, it's one of life's experiences I'd rather pass on. But I do believe that these periods of intense fright, especially those that make us aware of our own mortality, can give us a whole new perspective on life and our relationships with others. In a matter of a few short hours, we are forced to confront the uncomfortable reality that we will not be here forever. Time becomes a precious commodity. I am used to hearing patients voice all kinds of regrets in the CCU: Why did I allow myself to grow apart from my son or daughter? Why am I working in a job that I hate? Why don't I ever do anything for myself? When was the last time that I told my husband that I loved him? If we learn from this experience and make the necessary changes in our lives, the emotional toll exacted by the CCU can yield terrific dividends.

Depending on their progress and the number of patients waiting for their bed, most patients are out of the CCU within 24 to 36 hours. You will be kept in the CCU for a longer period if you're running a fever, still experiencing pain, have developed a dangerous arrhythmia, or are at risk of heart failure. Although some hospitals have special "step-down" units specifically designed for cardiac patients, most will simply move the stabilized patient to a regular medical floor. Leaving the CCU is a good sign. Although you're not completely out of the woods—for the first few days after a heart attack, there's always a danger of arrhythmia or even infection—the crisis is over.

There are some patients who never make it out of the CCU. Most often, the patient who doesn't survive has developed a fatal arrhythmia that has completely destroyed the normal pumping action of the heart. Fluid gathers in the heart and lungs. If a doctor listens with a stethoscope, she will hear an extra sound called a gallop, evidence that the heart is failing. If the damage to the heart is extensive, the patient may go into cardiogenic shock: The heart stops sending blood to the brain and the extremities, and the kidneys cease to function. Many of these patients will die. Fortunately, most of the time we are able to avert this kind of tragedy.

Chapter 16

THE ROAD
TO RECOVERY

AFTER even a brief stay in the protective environment of the CCU, many patients are startled when their floor nurse suggests that they sit in a chair instead of lying in their bed, or even that they try to walk unassisted to the bathroom. There was a time in the not-too-distant past when this would have been unheard of. When I first began practicing medicine, conventional wisdom dictated that heart attack patients with no other complications were to stay in bed for four weeks—no exceptions. Complications meant that an additional two weeks were tacked on to this sentence. It was believed that the heart needed complete rest to recuperate from the ordeal of a heart attack.

We now know that these periods of enforced bedrest may have caused more problems than they actually prevented. When you don't move, your muscles weaken. Your blood doesn't circulate properly, which can promote clots—exactly what you don't need after a heart attack. You can become constipated, depressed, and even suffer a certain amount of osteoporosis (thinning of the bones). In fact, according to an article published in the *American Journal of Nursing*, researchers estimate that the functional body loss after a mere three weeks of total bedrest is roughly equal to the effects of thirty years of aging! Thus, as soon as they're able patients are now encouraged to walk slowly—and I mean slowly—around the hospital corridors. Mild calisthenics—gently moving the arms and legs from a sitting position—may also be allowed. Each patient must have an exercise program that is individually tailored to her ability, gradually increasing the physical challenges as she gets stronger. There are a few patients who may need complete bedrest, and they are usually given a blood thinner, heparin, to prevent the formation of blood clots.

Although we encourage physical activity, this is not the time to test your limits or to prove anything to yourself or anybody else. The post–heart attack period is a critical time. For the next three months, your heart will be going through a lot of changes. Heart cells have died and scar tissue is forming. The work of the lost heart cells must be taken over by the surviving cells. Although you don't want to become an invalid, it's perfectly all right to indulge yourself a little. Don't expect to shift into high gear when you come home from the hospital. You will need more than your usual rest.

I have found that my women patients often have the most difficulty allowing someone else to cook for them or to clean. And most of all, they live in fear of becoming a burden on their families. But keep in mind that getting enough rest is just as important as taking your medication and keeping your doctor's appointments. Denying yourself a proper recovery period can be very short-sighted. Heart attacks can strike twice and often do.

Before you leave the hospital, your doctor will probably suggest that you take a modified exercise stress test. It is not a full stress test where you are exercised to your maximal heart beat—you won't be asked to do that until at least six weeks after your heart attack. In this "mini" stress test, you will be exercised up to about 120 beats per minute, the normal rate your heart would beat if you were walking up a flight of stairs or running across the house to answer the telephone. The purpose of the test is to assess your cardiac reserve, that is, to see if your heart can withstand the challenges of day-to-day living.

Even though it is not a real stress test, many patients are simply terrified at the mere thought of riding a bicycle or walking on a treadmill so soon after their heart attack. Their first instinct is to say no. Ironically, however, it is the patients who don't take the stress test who have the poorest prognosis. A recent landmark study from 11 leading medical centers showed that patients who either refuse to take the exercise stress test or can't because of continuing pain or heart failure die at a much higher rate than those who meet the challenge—willingly or unwillingly. There are probably many reasons for this. First, if a patient honestly feels incapable of surviving the test, she may actually be acutely and accurately aware of her own limitations. Second, the test provides the physician with important information. From it, she can assess how well the heart is pumping, and whether or not the patient is prone to arrhythmia during times of physical or emotional exertion. From this information, the physician can tailor an aftercare program to meet the patient's unique needs.

If a patient does very poorly on the stress test, the doctor may suggest cardiac catheterization to determine exactly where the problem is, and what, if anything, can be done about it. If the doctor believes that the patient cannot tolerate the exercise stress test, she can perform a drug-induced, or stress simulation, test by using drugs to dilate the arteries to see how the heart reacts during exertion. Although the exercise stress test is better, the simulated stress test provides at least some information as to how well the heart is performing.

I personally don't let a patient leave the hospital without giving her an echocardiogram to check the overall structure and function of her heart, as well as to see if there are any blood clots on the heart wall overlying the site of the damage that could break off and cause a stroke.

LEAVING THE HOSPITAL

During your hospital stay, a highly skilled team of doctors and nurses are hovering over you, practically monitoring your every breath on a 24-hour basis. While under their supervision, the staff makes sure that you're getting good care. You're on a strict low-fat, low-salt diet. You're forced to get enough rest, and you're not allowed to drink or smoke. In the highly rarified atmosphere of a hospital, the mundane worries of day-to-day living—the kids, the job, the car that has to go back to the body shop, and the pile of bills in your desk drawer—seem very remote. Friends, business associates, and even the most contentious of relatives usually refrain from arguing with you or telling you about things that might be upsetting.

Once you're out of the protective hospital setting, however, everything changes. For one thing, you will no longer be seeing your doctor every day. Your next appointment will probably be in two weeks. She may call you to check up on you, or you may call her in the case of an emergency or to ask specific questions, but she will no longer be there to provide daily reassurance. For another thing, you will no longer have a nursing staff at your disposal or the security of knowing that if something goes wrong the staff will be there to fix it. Whether you like it or not, you are now back in charge of your body.

Finally, once you're out of the hospital you're no longer isolated from the realities of life. You're soon preoccupied with family problems, earning a living, and even paying your medical bills. On top of that, you're probably deeply concerned about your health. Even if you have a very loving family and very supportive friends you will probably feel very much alone and even a bit frightened when you walk out of the hospital. After all, you are the one who had the heart attack—not your spouse or your best friend. You are the one who suffered the physical and emotional trauma that accompanies any life-threatening illness, but especially one that involves an organ as central to life as the heart. And you are the one who is terrified that it could happen again.

I have seen patients crippled by this fear, unable to take a few steps on their own or even engage in a lively conversation without worrying about dying. I don't tell these people not to worry. But I remind them that fear can be a powerful motivator, and if they can channel their nervous energy into working toward their recovery, they may find an inner strength that they never knew existed.

After a heart attack you may feel more vulnerable than you have ever felt in your entire life. As a doctor, I know that there is a lot more to be done after a heart attack than simply discharging the patient within the requisite seven to ten days and handing her a prescription for some medicine. Although we may have done our main job—saving a life—our work is just beginning. Now we must make sure that the patient has not merely survived but is able to maintain as good a quality of life as possible. To achieve this goal, before a heart attack patient leaves the hospital she and her doctor must sit down and work out a comprehensive aftercare program so that the patient feels confident in her ability to recover.

By the way, it takes two or more people to plan an aftercare program—it is not something that the doctor should do on her own. Simply handing a patient a sheet of paper outlining a diet and exercise plan is often counterproductive. To ensure compliance, a patient must not only know what to do but must understand why she's doing it. Therefore, a doctor has to be willing to devote enough time to teaching the post–heart attack patient how to maintain her own health. Unfortunately, the medical profession is often crisis-oriented: We're great in an emergency, but once the crisis has passed, we still tend to focus on the patient in the CCU rather than on the one who is stabilized and heading for recovery. I'm not saying that we should ignore our acutely ill patients, but we need to realize that time spent with a recovering patient is not any less important than time spent in the CCU. In fact, a small investment of time with a patient on the mend may actually help avert the next crisis.

A good aftercare plan consists of three major components: reviewing the patient's medical options; helping the patient make positive changes in her lifestyle, including an exercise and stress management program; and getting the patient to adhere to a diet tailored to her special needs.

MEDICAL OPTIONS

Following a heart attack, the patient and doctor must discuss her treatment options, including medication, and if warranted, surgery. Usually, the doctor will first try to put the patient on medication designed to dilate, or open up, the coronary arteries, such as nitroglycerine, to improve the blood flow to the heart. The patient may also require one or more medications including:

1. An antiarrhythmic medication such as Lidocaine or Quinidine
2. A cardiotonic drug such as digitalis, which strengthens and slows the contraction of the heart muscle and promotes the elimination of fluid from body tissues
3. An ACE inhibitor such as captopril to improve the contractility and pumping action of the heart

4. A beta blocker such as propranolol to control the sympathetic nervous system
5. A calcium channel blocker such as nifedipine to control coronary artery spasm and to lower blood pressure

In addition, the patient may be taking lipid-reducing drugs to cut cholesterol and/or antihypertensives to maintain a normal blood pressure. Because a patient is often under the care of several specialists, I have seen situations where one physician is unaware of the prescriptions being written by another. Cardiac drugs are strong drugs. Many interact poorly with each other. Side effects are not uncommon, especially in the case of some of the antiarrhythmic drugs and so-called cholesterol busters. Therefore, it is essential that you have a primary-care physician—either an internist or a cardiologist—who is serving as a traffic controller of sorts, monitoring the different medications that you are taking. All prescriptions should first be channeled through the primary-care doctor, who must watch the patient very carefully for any adverse reactions. There are computer programs your doctor can use to verify that the drugs you are taking will not interact harmfully. Ask her for a printout of this information.

If medication fails to do the job, the doctor may consider other alternatives that directly affect the coronary arteries, the precious lifeline that supplies the heart with vital oxygen and nutrients. If you want to keep the heart healthy, it's essential to keep the blood flowing freely through these arteries. As we discussed earlier, sometimes the right medication does the trick, and in those cases, the problem can be solved simply and noninvasively. But if the patient is still in pain, or not showing signs of improvement, the physician will probably consider two procedures that are a bit more complicated, but often yield spectacular results: balloon angioplasty and coronary artery bypass surgery.

Balloon Angioplasty

Since the rule of thumb in medicine is to do the easiest thing first, before opting for open-heart surgery we investigate whether the patient would be a good candidate for balloon angioplasty, also known as percutaneous transluminal coronary angioplasty (PTCA). Since its inception in the late 1970s, this ingenious procedure has virtually revolutionized the treatment of CAD, providing a simple solution to a complicated problem.

A guiding catheter with a small balloon on the end is inserted through an arm or leg to the place where the coronary is narrowed by obstruction. The balloon is then inflated, flattening the plaque against the artery wall, thus opening up the constricted artery. The balloon and the catheter are then removed, and if all is well, the blood flow is restored to the portion of the heart fed by that artery.

Angioplasty offers many advantages over open-heart surgery: It is relatively painless, far less traumatic, and can be performed with local anesthesia. As wonderful as it is, it is not for everyone. Angioplasty seems to be most successful in patients under sixty-five, and works better for men than for women. No one is sure why women don't do as well, except for the fact that women who have this procedure tend to be older than men and that female arteries are smaller and more difficult to work on. Newer and better designed angioplasty systems specifically tailored to women may offer some improvement in the future.

As a rule, people with diabetes, hypertension, and disease in several coronary arteries are usually not good candidates for angioplasty. Despite these shortcomings, most men and women who can have the procedure have good results. According to a national registry maintained by the National Institutes of Health, in 1988, about 90 percent of patients who underwent angioplasty were successful, an improvement of 30 percent over the last decade. However, 4 percent had prolonged angina, and as a result of angioplasty, they had to undergo emergency bypass. Sadly, 1 percent died either during the procedure or as a result of complications. Regardless of sex, within six months after the procedure, in about 25 percent of all cases, the artery became narrowed again. If that happens, the angioplasty can be redone, or bypass surgery may be required.

Angioplasty works best on small, discrete obstructions that are close to the aorta. It is most effective on plaque that is evenly distributed and is least effective on plaque that is heaped up on one side of the artery. The procedure is more dangerous if the lesion has calcified—a piece could break off and cause an obstruction in the vessel further down the line. Angioplasty is also more effective on some arteries than on others. For example, in most cases, doctors will choose bypass surgery over angioplasty if the left descending coronary artery is significantly blocked, because if that critical artery ceases to function, there is a high risk of sudden death.

The success rate of any new procedure—and certainly one as tricky as angioplasty, or as complicated as bypass—depends on the skill and experience of the physician at the helm and the quality of the hospital and staff backing her up. Before selecting a surgeon or cardiologist who will perform angioplasty, you and your doctor must carefully investigate the physician's credentials. As I often tell my patients, if you are considering balloon angioplasty, or any other surgical procedure, make sure that your physician has gotten her practice elsewhere. In a way, selecting a surgeon is a lot like buying a new car—you don't want to be the test driver.

If you are having angioplasty, check the cardiologist's credentials. In addition to three years of cardiology fellowship training, she should have a year of instruction that includes extensive angioplasty experience. Find out how many angioplasties she has performed, her overall success rate, as well as the number of mortalities and complications. You might also ask how many angioplasties she has successfully performed on women, and whether she feels that you personally are a good risk.

The hospital in which the procedure is performed should also have a backup surgical team on hand to do an emergency bypass if necessary. If something goes wrong, time is of the essence—you don't want to be carted halfway across town to another hospital. Nor do you want to be in a hospital where angioplasty is an exotic procedure—it should be done on a routine basis. Don't feel funny about asking a lot of questions about either the surgeon or the hospital: A good doctor will be forthcoming with her answers.

I personally seek out surgeons who fare better than the national average. For example, I recently referred a patient for angioplasty to a cardiologist who not only had an excellent reputation but who could back it up with a 95 percent success rate, no mortalities, and a scant 1.2 percent emergency-bypass rate. Granted, part of his high success rate might have been attributed to his ability to weed out the patients who would not be good angioplasty candidates, but I also feel that his superior skill is a major factor.

There are many advantages to balloon angioplasty over bypass surgery: It is quicker, easier, not nearly as traumatic, and it offers a better survival rate. But it doesn't always work and it can't be performed on everybody who needs it. For these patients, bypass surgery may be their only option.

Coronary Artery Bypass Grafting (CABG)

The left main coronary artery and the right coronary artery branch off from the aorta. The left main artery divides into branches called the left anterior descending anterior and the circumflex. The coronary arteries and their branches supply blood and oxygen to the heart. When one or more coronary arteries are blocked, and angioplasty has been ruled out, bypass surgery may be performed to ensure an adequate blood supply to the heart.

There are two methods of performing this procedure: In bypass surgery, a vein from another part of the body, usually the leg, is grafted or attached from the aorta to a point just downstream from the obstruction in the coronary artery, so the blood is detoured, or bypassed, around the blockage. Alternatively, one of the internal mammary arteries that runs inside the chest wall is freed up and inserted into the affected coronary artery, again just beyond the point of obstruction.

If possible, most surgeons today prefer to use the mammary artery over the leg vein because it is less painful for the patient during recovery and is less likely to become blocked itself as time goes on. However, the mammary procedure takes more time and is more difficult to perform than the one using the leg vein. In addition, it does not work as well on older patients. Since women are more likely to have emergency bypass surgery than men, they may not be good candidates for mammary artery grafts.

The decision to perform cardiac bypass surgery can only be made by a skilled surgeon and cardiologist following an angiogram that provides specific information about the anatomy of the coronary arteries. The team must consider several factors including the number of arteries affected, the location of the blockages, the overall health of the patient, and the results of other diagnostic procedures. As a rule of thumb, the more arteries that are narrowed or blocked, the greater the patient's risk of dying from a heart attack, and the more likely she is to benefit from surgery. The easiest vessels to operate on are those in which the obstruction is high up or close to the aorta.

The best results will be obtained on patients who suffer from chronic, debilitating angina: Studies show that 80 percent of these people will receive enormous relief from the pain after surgery. In addition, most patients with a 50 percent or more obstruction in their left main artery will probably benefit from bypass, since a heart attack resulting from a blockage of this critical artery will cut off blood to a major part of the heart, posing a serious risk. We also usually opt for surgery on someone with so-called three-vessel disease, characterized by blockages in the right coronary, the left anterior descending branch of the left artery, and the circumflex branch.

In sum, good candidates for bypass surgery are people whose lifestyle is being compromised by debilitating angina, or those who because of the number or location of their blockages run the greatest risk of sudden death in case of a heart attack. Judgment and experience are essential ingredients for a good decision. However, doctors are not infallible, and at times a second opinion may be necessary before the patient feels comfortable with proceeding with her doctor's recommendation.

More than 70 percent of all coronary bypass operations are performed on men. Women who have bypass surgery are usually older than men—a reflection of the fact that women develop CAD later in life—and are also sicker by the time of the operation. However, there may be other factors reflected in these statistics, including sex role stereotyping. A case in point: A recent study of 2,000 women bypass patients at Cedars Sinai Medical Center in Los Angeles suggested that doctors may be waiting too long to refer their women patients for surgery, ignoring symptoms in women they would have taken more seriously in men.

Bypass surgery is not without risk, especially for women. In fact, even the catheterization leading up to the procedure poses a real, albeit minimal, risk of which patients should be aware. During the catheterization, 1 out of 500 patients will suffer a heart attack, stroke, or other serious complication. During the bypass operation, 2 percent of all patients will die, and anywhere from 5 percent to 10 percent of all patients will have heart attacks either on the operating table or immediately following the surgery. Unfortunately, the prognosis for women is somewhat worse than for men. In fact, according to the Cedars Sinai study, women are twice as likely to die from the procedure as men. The fact that women are older and sicker when they have the surgery may be more of a factor in the mortality rate than sex. Also similar to angioplasty, the smaller size of the female arteries and heart might make it more difficult for the surgeon to perform the procedure.

Bypass surgery is major surgery. It can take several hours to perform, during which time the work of the heart is taken over by a mechanical heart-lung machine. Despite the rather arduous procedure, there are no guarantees that the bypass graft will remain clear. In fact, about 4 percent of all grafts will become clogged with plaque within the first year, and within ten years about 70 percent of all grafts will become closed and the operation will have to be performed again. However, some short-term studies show that patients who adhere to very low-cholesterol diets along with exercise and stress reduction programs may do better. Only time will tell if these patients continue to beat the odds.

After the surgery, recovery can take several months, although many patients say it takes a full year before they feel quite like themselves again. And some never do. A handful of studies suggest that women may experience more depression and sexual dysfunction than men postsurgery. However, it's not uncommon for both men and women to suffer from depression months or even years after the operation. We're not sure why, but a recent study may shed some light on the subject. Researchers monitored a group of bypass patients in nine medical centers in the United States, West Germany, Italy, Finland, Brazil, and Colombia. A year after the surgery, 20 percent of those patients were still depressed, and more importantly, 17 percent of the group suffered from a subtle form of impaired mental ability. They had difficulty learning new information, concentrating on any one subject for a long period of time, and performing certain mental tasks as quickly as they did before surgery.

Doctors participating in the study speculate that some of the mental problems may stem from the surgical procedure itself. For instance, when the work of the heart is being performed by the heart-lung machine, the brain may not get enough oxygen, and therefore it may become slightly damaged. Another theory is that during surgery the blood may form tiny clots that could cause several small, undetectable strokes.

Many doctors have criticized this study, noting that years of oxygen deprivation caused by CAD could also yield similar results—in other words, the disease, not the cure, is to blame. Obviously, more studies must be done in this area before we can conclusively say that bypass surgery is the culprit, but until then it's important to factor in the possibility of depression or minimal mental impairment when weighing the risks versus benefits of this potentially lifesaving surgery.

Friends and relatives of bypass patients and the patients themselves should be aware of the fact that after surgery the patient will not only require physical care but will need tremendous emotional support to help her mend properly. On this point, women are at a distinct disadvantage. Often, after a man has bypass surgery he returns home to a wife and family that typically have reorganized the household to meet his needs. However, women as a group are widowed earlier in life than men, therefore very often when a woman bypass patient is ready to leave the hospital she returns to an empty house where she must fend for herself. A woman who is living alone must be given special attention during this vulnerable time and must make it a point to reach out to her friends and loved ones. If possible, she should arrange for a friend or relative to stay with her for a week or two following her release from the hospital. I also recommend that bypass patients—especially those who are alone—join a patient support group such as Mended Hearts, which will give them an opportunity to meet others who have had a similar experience. The hospital staff can refer you to a group near you, or you can contact Mended Hearts directly.

Despite the risks and possible complications of bypass surgery, many people who have had the operation now enjoy a vastly improved quality of life. The mortality statistics are scary and the risk of having a heart attack or stroke on the operating table is cause for concern, but nevertheless, I believe there are some risks that are well worth taking. I have seen people so debilitated by angina that they literally can't take a few steps without feeling pain and becoming out of breath. Others face certain premature death if they do not have any surgical therapy. If all the other possibilities have been exhausted, and you are faced with the prospect of living a very limited existence or are at risk for sudden or premature death due to CAD, I certainly believe that the option of bypass surgery should be thoroughly investigated.

Heart Transplants

If the heart has suffered irreparable damage due to disease, neither drugs nor surgery may be effective treatments. The only option left is a heart transplant: replacing the sick heart with a healthy, donor heart. Despite its rocky start in 1968, when mortality for transplants was so high that most medical facilities stopped performing them, today about 1,700 of these procedures are done annually. Heart transplants today are a lot safer: Patients have about a 50 percent chance of survival for five years following the surgery. Many more transplants would be performed if there were more donor hearts available, but donors are few and far between. A donor must be under forty years old, and has to have died from an injury that in no way adversely affected the heart. Even if the medical facility locates a likely donor, it is still difficult getting family members to agree to the donation if their loved one did not specifically will his organs to an organ bank. For more information about transplants, talk to your cardiologist.

RETURNING TO LIFE

The physician must help the patient honestly reassess her lifestyle to determine what, if anything, may have contributed to the heart attack. If I have a patient who is under a great deal of stress, at work or at home, we discuss various ways that she can either eliminate the stress or learn how to better cope with it. I believe very strongly that in times of difficulty, such as the post–heart attack period, short-term psychotherapy can be very helpful for the patient and her family. For example, I recently had a patient whose blood pressure would rise at the mere mention of her fifteen-year-old daughter, who was going through typical teenage rebellion. As part of her aftercare program, I insisted that she and her daughter see a family counselor to improve their deteriorating relationship.

After a few counseling sessions, I saw a tremendous change in both of them. The daughter became a real and valuable resource during her mother's recuperative period, often cooking meals and assisting with housework. In fact, my patient was so impressed by her daughter's display of responsibility that she voluntarily gave in on some issues that had nearly brought them to blows in the past. I can't say for sure whether therapy was totally responsible for improving this relationship, or that it helped prevent a second heart attack, but I do believe it contributed greatly to improving the stressful atmosphere in that household, thus diminishing what had been a significant danger to my patient's health.

Although I believe that it's important to reduce unnecessary stress after a heart attack, I do not believe that heart attack survivors are too fragile to deal with emotions. Unfortunately, some patients believe that any form of excitement—good or bad—will result in another attack. This can be extremely frustrating for their family and friends. For example, I recently got a call from a patient's college-age son who complained that since his mother's heart attack six months earlier they have been unable to have a meaningful conversation. "Every time I try to talk to her about anything important to me, or disagree with anything that she says, she tells me that I shouldn't say things that upset her. Am I being selfish for wanting to include her in what's going on in my life?"

I quickly assured the son that he wasn't doing anything wrong. Despite her heart attack, his mother is still a member of the family and should be treated as one. Contrary to popular belief, a heart attack does not leave its victim in a weakened state for life, nor will every emotional or physical stress have a devastating effect on the healed heart. In fact, just the opposite is true. I like to remind my patients that once the healing period is over, the newly formed scar tissue is actually stronger than the original heart muscle and every bit as resilient. Although everyone should take good care of themselves after a heart attack, it is important to try to live as normal a life as possible. It is not necessary or even appropriate for someone to use heart disease as a shield against all of life's problems, nor is it right to allow a family member to crawl into a hole and hide from the world.

This is not to say that living under chronic stress is harmless. There is a real difference, however, between a family that has periodic disagreements and one that is constantly bickering. For everyone's health and sanity, it is important for family members to learn to communicate without sniping at each other. The family that comes to blows during every discussion needs to learn how to relate to each other in a more constructive manner. If family members can't do it on their own, professional intervention may be necessary.

Sometimes a patient may truly feel vulnerable during times of intense emotion, especially if she is prone to angina. In this case, I might advise the patient to take nitroglycerine before discussing a difficult issue, but I would rarely advise someone to pretend the problem wasn't there. Keep in mind that hidden anger and hostility can be much more lethal than anger that is out in the open, and it can wreak havoc on your relationships with others as well as on your own health.

Sometimes it is not the patient who avoids stress at all cost but an over-protective husband who won't let his wife resume her normal life. After a wife has a heart attack, the husband often becomes completely consumed with fear that his spouse will die, and as a result, he tries to shield her from the world. A case in point is Margaret, a patient of mine who before her heart attack was a vital, independent woman with a very active life. For fifteen years, Margaret always came to my office by herself, but after her heart attack her husband Jim chauffeured her back and forth to her appointments and anywhere else she had to go.

I noticed that Margaret was getting more and more depressed and I suspected that Jim's constant hovering was beginning to get her down. During one of her appointments, Margaret confessed that Jim never let her out of his sight. Furthermore, he had instructed their married children not to trouble her with family problems or to ask her to babysit for fear that it would be too much for her. Margaret said that she desperately longed for some time alone or the chance to meet a friend for lunch. Most of all, she missed honest conversations with her children and taking care of her grandchildren.

At that point, I invited Jim in from the waiting room and gently told him that although Margaret was doing well physically, I was worried about her emotional state. I stressed that if he truly loved his wife and wanted her to fully recover he had to let her resume a normal life. That meant letting her go places by herself, allowing her to have uncensored conversations with her children, and even permitting her to babysit for her grandchildren if she wished. Although it took some convincing, Jim agreed to give Margaret the space she required and I believe she is healthier for it.

It's also important to remember that a heart attack doesn't just happen to one person. Its effect is felt by an entire family. Any parental illness can have a devastating effect on children who are bound to feel frightened, depressed, and even angry. Don't forget to explain to your children exactly what happened—their fantasies may be worse than the reality—and let them know that with good medical care and a lot of love even someone who has had a heart attack can lead a normal life with a normal life span. When under stress, even the best of parents can lash out and say hurtful things, so be extra careful not to make children feel guilty or responsible for your illness.

After a heart attack, some patients seek counseling to help them clarify aspects of their lives of which they may be unsure. Although some patients may be eager to return to work, there are many others who may feel the need to make a career change, especially if they're in high-stress, low-satisfaction jobs. In fact, if it weren't for their heart attack, I believe many of these people would have continued on the same occupational treadmill, year after year, never allowing themselves the luxury of introspection or the right to reexamine their lives. The heart attack was the catalyst that shocked them out of their complacency, and in that respect it may have actually been a blessing in disguise.

If a woman has devoted her life to being a caregiver, a heart attack may be an especially devastating blow. For the first time in her life, she is going to have to accept help. When I encounter a patient who is resistant to the notion of asking her family for support, it is often because she is completely out of touch with her own needs. For decades, everyone in her household had come first. She has simply forgotten how to think of herself in a healthfully selfish manner. And until she can, she will never be truly well.

Before I allow these women to leave the hospital, I give them a special assignment. I ask them to compose a wish list of everything in life that they want for themselves—not for their husbands, or their kids, or their parents, or their siblings; just for themselves. For many of these women, this exercise is excruciatingly difficult. Sometimes they'll spend days staring at a blank page before they are able to make the first entry. But once they begin to focus clearly on their own aspirations, many of them never want to stop. I really believe that this exercise can have a profound effect on a woman's life, whether or not she's had a heart attack. But for a woman whose health is in peril, learning to care about herself is an important first step in learning how to take better care of herself.

SEX AFTER A HEART ATTACK

For many people, making love is a life-affirming act; this may be especially true for women who have had a heart attack. A heart attack is a brutal reminder that your body won't last forever. It can make the strongest person feel frightened and helpless. It can be a devastating blow that can rob even the most confident, optimistic woman of her self-esteem. Often, the resumption of sexual relations can help restore the confidence she may have lost—not just confidence in the ability of her heart to keep on beating during a state of sexual arousal but confidence in her own ability to be sexy, attractive, and desirable. Thus, the transition from patient to lover is an important milestone in a woman's recovery.

After a heart attack, I sit down with every one of my patients and have a frank discussion about sex. I think every doctor should. Many patients have a great deal of fear and many misconceptions about sex. They may believe that the excitement of an orgasm could be lethal to their heart, but nothing could be further from the truth. Most patients will be able to withstand the rigors of normal sexual activity within a month or so after leaving the hospital. The rule of thumb is that if you are capable of running up two flights of stairs without experiencing pain or undue stress, you will be able to resume sexual intercourse.

Although some patients may require more time before they feel physically or emotionally ready, I have yet to tell a cardiac patient to refrain from all sexual activity for the rest of her life. I have, however, encountered patients who may want to. Their lack of sexual desire is often due to the depressing effect of certain medications, especially if they are taking beta blockers. In these cases, I either try to reduce the dose or change the medication.

When you do resume sexual activity, it's important to begin slowly and easily, gradually working your way up to your normal sexual pattern. Think of it this way: If you were training to run the Boston Marathon, you wouldn't do the whole 26 miles the first time out. You would probably try to run a few blocks at a time, slowly building up your endurance. The same is true for sex. You may find that you tire easily in the beginning, and even may have to stop and catch your breath along the way. But you can take heart in knowing that in time you will return to normal.

Although I encourage patients to resume sexual relations as soon as they can, I recognize that not all relationships are the same. For some couples, sex may be a beautiful expression of love and a source of mutual comfort. For others, the bedroom may be more of a battleground where one partner attempts to dominate and control the other. In these cases, one or both partners may be so demanding that sexual interludes may seem more like an endless marathon than making love. Although I don't want to judge the quality of a relationship, it is my job to protect the health of my patient. In cases where sex is very stressful, I do advise couples to alter their sexual styles, especially during the critical recovery period.

In other types of relationships, otherwise loving partners may enjoy the excitement of a good, heated argument before kissing and making up. The romantic in me can certainly understand the benefit of these theatrics, but the doctor in me says, "Hey, wait a minute. Every time you fight your sympathetic nervous system starts shooting off beta agonists that are going to constrict your blood vessels and make your heart work harder. Do you really want to do this before you have sex?" And the answer is no. After a heart attack, sex provides enough of a cardiac workout by itself, but if it's accompanied by a rush of negative emotions it could place too great a burden on the healing heart. Your best bet is to approach sex in a happy, relaxed state of body and mind.

Many patients have asked me whether extramarital affairs are too stressful after a heart attack. There is no evidence that affairs by themselves are responsible for heart attacks. In fact, some relationships outside of marriage may be a lot less stressful than those in wedlock. But if the affair involves a great deal of subterfuge—if you live in fear of your spouse or his spouse or both families finding out—or if the relationship itself is tension-provoking, then it could be detrimental to your health.

How do you determine if a relationship—within marriage or outside of it—is too stressful? Unfortunately, your doctor can't do it for you. You are the only one who can accurately assess the quality of your relationships, and whether or not they are heart-healthy. Your doctor can help by listening to what you have to say and by helping you sort out your feelings. In some cases, your doctor may refer you and/or your partner for psychological counseling. At times, even a sex therapist may be consulted to help a couple work out their difficulties.

Not every woman who leaves the hospital is ready to slip on a negligee and hop into bed with her spouse or lover. In fact, many are so devastated by the heart attack that they don't want to even think about sex, let alone talk about it. It's almost as if these women are in mourning, but they are not merely grieving over the loss of their youth. Heart attacks usually occur at the same time when things begin to change in a woman's body—and often these changes are perceived negatively. Our faces begin to wrinkle, our hair becomes gray, and our breasts begin to sag. The heart attack is just one more insult to our already vulnerable psyche.

After the heart attack, some women seem to surrender their sexual identity altogether, opting out of the sexual arena. They lose interest in their appearance, make no attempt to maintain their weight, and neither look nor feel attractive. When I see this starting to happen, I try to intervene early on to stop this downward spiral before it becomes a permanent way of life. Although it's not easy to help these women turn their life around, small but positive steps in the right direction—a weekly exercise class or even a trip to the hairdresser—can help restore their confidence.

Before you leave the hospital, it may take several months for you to feel like your old self again. You're badly shaken, scared, and exhausted. Everybody is. But within a short time, your body will mend, your heart will pump as strongly as ever before, and soon, you may want to forget about the whole ordeal altogether. But don't. If you pretend that the heart attack never happened, you could be missing out on the opportunity of a lifetime. In many cases, a heart attack is a warning sign. Something in your life or lifestyle has inflicted a mortal wound to your heart. Your heart, the marvelous, resilient organ that it is, has adjusted to the blow and has not given up. Now it's your turn to do everything in your power to protect the portion of your heart that is still alive and beating, because it cannot survive without your help.

VII

TAKING CARE
OF YOURSELF

❧

Chapter 17

WORKING WITH
YOUR DOCTOR

IF you ask a woman to make a list of the ten most important people in her life, I seriously doubt that she would include her doctor. To most women, doctors are to be seen only when absolutely necessary, such as during illness or pregnancy. Therefore, for women who are feeling fine and who are not pregnant, two or three or more years can slip between visits. I believe very strongly that when it comes to their own medical care, women—especially women under forty—are shortchanging themselves. A doctor should not just be someone you call to get a prescription or to deliver a baby. A doctor should be an integral part of your life. Your doctor should be someone who knows you as a person, not just as a sick person.

Every woman over eighteen who values her health should have an annual physical exam performed by a competent internist or primary-care physician. These two types of practitioners are specially trained in general adult patient care. Often, women fall prey to what I call the "body parts" approach to medicine. When they do see a doctor, they usually only see a gynecologist, which I feel is a mistake. This is not to say that gynecology is unimportant. I am not criticizing specialists. Although I personally take a "holistic" approach to the practice of medicine, I often refer patients to specialists myself. By definition, however, the role of the specialist is to monitor a particular organ system. And because a woman's body consists of much more than breasts, ovaries, and a uterus, she needs to be examined annually by a physician whose primary job is to evaluate her overall health.

There are many reasons the annual physical is important, but one of the most important is that it will enable you to develop a relationship with your doctor. If your doctor is familiar with your family medical history, your lifestyle, and your overall health, she will be in a better position to detect small problems before they blossom into big ones. Second, if you have a good rapport with your doctor, you will be more likely to pick up the phone and let her know if you're experiencing any unusual symptoms. I believe that if more women felt comfortable with their doctors, there would be fewer women ignoring important symptoms such as chest pain, and there would be fewer cases of unreported heart attacks among women. Getting to know your doctor is well worth the investment: One day, it might save your life.

The annual examination should never be rushed: Both the patient and the doctor must be willing to invest the time and energy to ensure that the patient's examination is thorough. Some doctors may not want to spend the necessary time to do this, and some patients may be more than willing to let their doctor off the hook because they themselves don't want to risk learning anything unpleasant or threatening. But that is not good medicine and neither party is serving the best interest of the patient. Below is a discussion of important aspects of the physical examination.

THOROUGH FAMILY/PERSONAL MEDICAL HISTORY

Ideally, this information should be taken the first time a patient visits a new doctor and it should be updated during each subsequent visit. To facilitate the process, I advise patients to come prepared. Your doctor should ask you about any illnesses, such as rheumatic fever or high blood pressure during a past pregnancy, that could make you more prone to cardiovascular problems down the road. Also, anticipate that your doctor is going to ask you about any close relatives (parents, grandparents, siblings, or children) who have either died from heart disease or currently have heart disease, high blood pressure, diabetes, high cholesterol, or a congenital heart problem. Make sure that your doctor knows if you are under a great deal of stress, or if you have a history of either alcohol or drug abuse.

If the doctor suspects a problem, the patient must also be willing to agree to any reasonable diagnostic testing that her doctor may feel is necessary. I know that some tests may be uncomfortable, expensive (depending on your insurance), and often downright anxiety-provoking. But if your doctor feels that further testing is important to verify a diagnosis, I believe it is the patient's obligation to give serious consideration to the doctor's request.

The first meeting with a new doctor is a very important one, and one for which you should come well prepared. Your job is to provide valuable information about your family and personal medical history. Your doctor's job is to record this information, and put it in the context of your life. Any good doctor should be willing to devote at least one full hour to a new patient. (I have found that in most cases even that is not enough time.) I usually begin the interview by asking the patient about her birthplace, schooling, family, job, and other general aspects of her life. This conversa-

PHYSICAL EXAMINATION

WEIGHT	HEIGHT	TEMP	PULSE	RESP	BLOOD PRESSURE

GENERAL APPEARANCE

SKIN   HAIR

HEAD

EYES

EARS

NOSE & THROAT

NECK   BREASTS

THORAX

LUNGS

HEART

ABDOMEN

                                          HERNIA

GENITALIA

RECTAL

EXTREMITIES

LYMPH NODES

NEUROLOGICAL

		PRL	BI	TR	ABD	CR	K–J	A–J	PLTRS
R									
L									

SPECIAL EXAMS	LABORATORY	
	HEMOGL	SEGS
	RBC	STABS
	WBC	EOS
	HCT	BAS
INITIAL IMPRESSION	MCHC	LYMP
	MCV	MONO
	CSR	
	URINE – COLOR	
	SP G	
TREATMENT OR DIAGNOSTIC PLAN	MICRO	
	REACT	
	SUGAR	
	ALBUMIN	

8103

MEDICAL HISTORY

NAME		AGE	SEX	S M D W
ADDRESS		PHONE		DATE
SPONSOR	ADDRESS			
OCCUPATION	REF BY		ACKN	

CHIEF COMPLAINT

PRESENT ILLNESS

HISTORY — MILITARY

— SOCIAL

— FAMILY

— MARITAL

— MENSTRUAL	MENARCHE		PARA			L M P		X		X		X

— ILLNESS	MEASLES	MUMPS	PERT	VAR	PNEU	PLEUR	TYPH	MAL	RH FEV	SC FEV	DIPHTH

OTHER

— TRAUMA. SURGERY

REVIEW OF SYSTEMS

HEAD

EYES

EARS

NOSE & THROAT

NECK

BREASTS

CARDIO — RESPIRATORY

GASTRO — INTESTINAL

GENITO — URINARY

V. D.

MUSCULO — SKELETAL

SKIN

ALLERGY

NEURO — PSYCH

tion sets the stage for me: It places a patient in a framework and sketches in the broad outlines of her daily life.

I then take a comprehensive medical history. We cover not only the reason for which she came to me but review all aspects of her health, any past illnesses or operations, her family's health, and I get some idea of her personal habits and important relationships. After that, when I feel that the patient is comfortable with me, I begin the physical examination. Although every doctor probably has a slightly different approach, the following outline reviews the basic points that should be covered during a thorough physical. (On pages 191 and 192 is a copy of a standardized examination form that is used by many physicians.)

After taking the height and weight of the patient, the four vital signs are recorded: temperature, heart rate, respiratory rate, and blood pressure. The last should be taken in both arms, and while the patient is lying down, sitting up, and standing. Next, the four sets of orifices of the head are examined: I look into the eyes, ears, nose, and mouth of the patient, using special instruments to do so. The neck is next examined with the hands and with the stethoscope, and I assess for signs of obstruction in the great blood vessels of the brain. I check the state of the thyroid gland in the front of the neck and I begin the search for enlarged lymph nodes. These are checked in the neck, above the collar bones, in the arm pits, above the elbows, and in the groin. The chest, including the breasts and the heart, are examined next, followed by the abdominal examination. The external genitalia and a rectal examination, with a test for blood in the patient's stool, are next. Finally, a brief but comprehensive neurological examination finishes the first comprehensive examination.

LABORATORY WORKUP

Your doctor should order a series of laboratory tests that include:

1. A lipid profile to check your overall cholesterol level, as well as the HDL/LDL ratio and total triglycerides. (Ideally, if you are without any risk factor for CAD, total cholesterol should be less than 239, HDL should be higher than 40, and triglycerides should be less than 190.)
2. A complete blood count (CBC) to measure red blood cell count or hematocrit. (A higher-than-normal value increases your risk of heart attack or stroke, while a lower-than-normal value suggests anemia.)
3. Analysis of a blood sample to show that your liver and kidneys are working well and that you do not lack essential minerals, including iron.
4. A urinalysis to rule out infection or early kidney disease.

5. An annual Pap test for uterine cancer. In this painless procedure a sample of cells secreted by the uterus are gathered by the physician during the pelvic examination and sent to a laboratory for analysis. This test should be performed on all women age eighteen or older, and on younger women if they are sexually active.

MAMMOGRAM

If you are between thirty-five and thirty-nine, your doctor will probably send you for a mammogram or X ray of the breasts for early detection of cancer. If the mammogram is normal, it should be repeated every two years after age forty, and annually after age fifty. (If a woman is at high risk of developing breast cancer—that is, a close relative has it—she may be referred for a mammogram earlier or more frequently.)

ELECTROCARDIOGRAM

I believe that every woman over forty should have an electrocardiogram, or EKG, as part of her annual physical. This painless, noninvasive test will show whether her heart has sustained any damage due to oxygen deprivation or whether her heartbeat is regular. An EKG is the only way to tell whether a patient may have had silent heart attack—death of heart muscle without her even knowing it. Since more than one-third of all heart attacks in women go unreported, I feel that this test is critical. For a more thorough description of the EKG, see page 152.

OTHER POSSIBLE TESTS

If you are at high risk for acquired immune deficiency syndrome (AIDS), that is, if you use intravenous drugs, have had sex with a carrier of the virus, or engage in unsafe sex outside of a long-term, monogamous relationship, your physician may recommend an AIDS test.

CHOOSING A DOCTOR

If you don't have an internist or primary-care physician, there are several ways you can go about finding one:

1. Ask a friend who is particularly happy with her medical care for the name of her physician. However, keep in mind that simply because a

friend recommends a doctor it doesn't mean that you will like her. If possible, see if you can make an appointment to meet with the doctor. Depending on office policy, some doctors will schedule a brief meeting free of charge with a prospective patient.

2. Call your county medical society. Most counties in the United States have medical societies that will provide you with the names of three physicians in your area.

3. Call your local hospital. The Department of Internal Medicine at your local hospital or medical school may provide the names of physicians with whom they are affiliated.

4. Contact the American Society of Internal Medicine. This professional organization will provide you with a list of board-certified internists in your area. Call or write:

American Society of Internal Medicine
1101 Vermont Ave., NW
Washington, DC 20005
Tel. 202/289-1700

5. If you have a name of a physician and you want to check out her credentials, you can request an AMA physician profile from the American Medical Association in Chicago. The profile will tell you where she went to medical school, where she is licensed to practice medicine, and which, if any, are her specialties. To request an AMA physician profile write:

American Medical Association
535 North Dearborn St.
Chicago, IL 60610

6. In addition, in the reference section of most libraries, there are physicians directories compiled by the county medical societies and the AMA. For information, ask your librarian.

WHAT TO EXPECT FROM YOUR DOCTOR

Future visits to your doctor may not be as comprehensive as your first, but they should not be superficial either. Before you arrive, your doctor should review your file so that she is familiar with your case. It's reasonable to expect your doctor to know who you are, what problems she has treated you for in the past, and what medication you are taking. If your doctor makes no attempt to get to know you, I feel that you should make it your business to get to know another doctor.

It's also within your rights to expect your doctor to return your phone calls as quickly as she can. In my experience, few patients call a doctor unless they really need to, and therefore I make it a point to call everyone back as soon as I get a free moment. It is also reasonable to expect your doctor to be there for you during a crisis, such as a heart attack. I personally feel that it is inexcusable to send a patient to the hospital and not to be there for her, unless you are tied up in another emergency.

A woman must be comfortable enough with her doctor to speak openly about private details of her life that could affect her health. She should also feel that her doctor is not there just to treat a physical problem but is someone she can turn to for help during times of emotional crises.

It is also critical to have a doctor who you feel takes you seriously and doesn't dismiss any of your symptoms or questions without proper investigation. As I've noted earlier in this book, studies show that doctors may be ignoring the early warning signs of CAD in women, and may not be referring women for diagnostic testing in a timely fashion. Whether you are experiencing chest pain or any other complaint, it is important for your doctor to try to determine the cause of your problem. In some cases, you may require further diagnostic testing. However, in other cases, your doctor may feel that she can make a diagnosis based solely on symptoms and history. At the very least, you should feel that your doctor has given careful thought and consideration to your case. If the problem has not improved, or if you're dissatisfied with your doctor's explanation, you may need to seek a second opinion.

As a physician, I set a high standard for myself and I feel that most other doctors do the same. As good as we may try to be, it's important for patients to remember that doctors are not infallible. A good doctor will try to be a competent, caring physician, but even the best of doctors can make mistakes. If you're looking for a perfect doctor, you'll never find one. But if you have realistic expectations, you will find a doctor who is good enough for the job, and who with your help can be an excellent resource.

WHAT EVERY WOMAN NEEDS TO KNOW AND WHEN SHE NEEDS TO KNOW IT

AGES TWO TO SEVENTEEN

Every girl should have an annual physical examination by her pediatrician that includes the following:

1. Her growth patterns should be monitored.
2. Her blood pressure should be measured.

3. A CBC (complete blood count) should be performed.
4. If a sibling, parent, or grandparent has a cholesterol level in the ninety-fifth percentile, the child should have a lipid profile. If her total cholesterol is less than 150 and her HDL is higher than 40, the test need not be repeated for five years.
5. If she is sexually active, she should have a Pap test.

AGES EIGHTEEN TO TWENTY-NINE

1. By age eighteen, every woman should have an annual physical with an internist.
2. A Pap test and a complete pelvic exam should be done during her annual physical.
3. By age twenty, every woman should have at the very least a screening test to determine total blood cholesterol. If the level is more than 240 mg/dl, she should have a complete blood lipid profile to determine HDL–LDL breakdown and triglycerides.
4. If a woman takes oral contraceptives, she should have a lipid profile done annually.

AGES THIRTY TO THIRTY-NINE

1. As part of her annual physical, by age thirty every woman should have a complete blood lipid profile. If it is within normal range, it need not be repeated for five years. However, if she has any risk factors for CAD (family history, obesity, smoking, etc.) it should be redone every two years. If a woman takes oral contraceptives, the lipid profile should be done annually.
2. A Pap test and pelvic exam should be done annually.
3. Between ages thirty-five and thirty-nine she should have a baseline mammogram. If the mammogram is normal, it can be redone every two years. If she has a family history of breast cancer, her physician may recommend it more often.

AGES FORTY TO FORTY-NINE

1. As part of her complete physical, by age forty a woman should have an electrocardiogram (EKG) every year.
2. Every two years, she should have a mammogram.
3. A Pap test and a pelvic examination should be done each year.
4. Every year she should have a blood lipid profile.

AGE FIFTY AND OLDER

By age fifty, the following tests should be performed annually:

1. Mammogram
2. Lipid profile
3. EKG
4. Pap test

Chapter 18

GOOD NEWS
FOR WOMEN
ABOUT EXERCISE

STUDIES show that about 90 percent of all women don't exercise regularly and that as many as 17 percent (nearly twice as many as men) are completely inactive—that is, they never exercise. In fact, 90 percent of all people who begin exercise programs eventually quit. Fitness experts say that women in particular are intimidated by the macho approach of many of today's popular exercise gurus. The majority of women who don't exercise regularly simply can't identify with the minority of "superfit" women—such as marathon winners or body builders—who discuss their grueling dawn-to-dusk fitness routines on talk shows or produce their own exercise videos. When women do venture into health clubs or read one of the many popular books on exercise, they are often turned off by jargon such as target heart rate (optimum heart rate during exercise) and VO_2 max (measurement of how the body utilizes oxygen). Discouraged, the average woman believes that exercise isn't for her.

Here's some good news for every woman who has ever squandered money on a health club membership that she has never used, or invested in a stack of exercise videos that she has never played. You don't have to burn with Jane Fonda or pump iron with Cher to get maximum benefit out of an exercise program. New research shows that a little bit of exercise goes a long way toward achieving good health in women. In fact, by just walking 30 minutes a day, you can reduce your risk of dying from heart disease by 50 percent!

The Institute for Aerobics Research and the Cooper Clinic in Dallas followed more than 13,000 men and women for an average of eight years to see if physical fitness levels correlated with death rates. Based on the results of an exercise treadmill test, the group was divided into five levels of fitness ranging from the most fit to the least fit. As might be expected, the women in the least fit group had the highest mortality rate (39.5 women per 10,000) and the women in the most fit group had the lowest (8.5 per 10,000). Women in the second lowest fitness group had nearly half the death rate (20.5 per 10,000) than that of women in the least fit group. In fact, these women experienced the biggest health gain of any other group in the study! Graduating from the least fit category to the next fit category did not entail anything but going from a completely sedentary lifestyle to one that included a brisk walk for at least a half hour every day. These women did not have to join a gym or jog religiously to achieve these dramatic results. All they had to do was add moderate amounts of physical activity to their otherwise inactive lives.

According to the study's leader, Steven N. Blair, PED, of the Institute of Aerobics Research, the half-hour walk doesn't have to be done all at once. You can walk for 10 or 15 minutes at a time and still experience a significant reduction in risk for heart disease. In fact, Dr. Blair is adamant that any increase in activity level that makes you less sedentary will help prevent heart disease. In other words, every time you walk up a flight of stairs, walk a few blocks, or do some light gardening you are reducing your risk of having a heart attack.

Studies such as this one prove that exercise is powerful medicine. Without it, we cannot perform at peak efficiency. Our muscles need to push and pull to maintain their strength. Our lungs need to be exercised by periods of rapid expansion and contraction, and our hearts need to be challenged by spurts of physical activity that make them beat harder and faster for short intervals.

We know for a fact that exercise helps control some of the risk factors for CAD. Moderate amounts of exercise (such as walking a half hour a day at 3–4 mph) can do the following:

1. Decrease blood pressure
2. Reduce triglyceride levels (high blood triglycerides are a leading risk factor for heart disease in women)
3. Help control obesity by burning up calories
4. Raise HDL in premenopausal women (but not in postmenopausal women)
5. Provide a good outlet for stress

Some scientists claim that exercise actually promotes the growth of blood vessels delivering blood to the heart. Therefore, they say that it directly prevents the heart from experiencing oxygen deprivation that would lead to a myocardial infarction. But as of yet there is no hard scientific evidence to prove this theory. We do know, however, that certain forms of exercise appear to have a beneficial effect on how the heart works.

The heart is a muscle, and like other muscles, it needs to be exercised to stay fit. When you are inactive, your heartbeat slows down. When you take a brisk walk, your heartbeat increases. The body's metabolism speeds up. The heart and lungs must work harder to meet the increased demand for oxygen. The more you exercise, the more the heart and lungs become accustomed to the increased workload. The heart is able to put out more blood per single stroke than it was when it was deconditioned—that is, it is able to do more work with less effort. The muscles learn to extract oxygen from the cells more efficiently.

The heart, lungs, and other body organs also perform their jobs better. As a result, during times of rest the well-exercised heart is able to meet the body's normal demands with ease. The resting heart rate drops, an indication that the heart is able to accomplish the same tasks with less exertion. Exercise builds up stamina, which comes in handy during times of stress. If the conditioned heart is suddenly called upon to do extra work—for example, if the blood pressure suddenly rises—the heart should be able to meet the challenge well. This ability of the heart to cope with a sudden increase in workload is called cardiac reserve. People who exercise regularly usually have more cardiac reserve than sedentary people whose heart is unaccustomed to hard work. Exercise is also especially important for women because it strengthens bones and muscles, providing protection against osteopororis.

GETTING STARTED: A WALKING PROGRAM FOR THE NOVICE

If you have CAD or have had a heart attack, turn to page 205. If you are over thirty-five and have been sedentary, do not start any exercise program without first consulting with your doctor. Although most people can exercise safely, some people—especially those with hidden cardiac problems—cannot. In fact, there is a real risk of sudden death for anyone who undertakes a vigorous exercise program without proper preparation. Based on your risk factors and general state of health, your doctor will decide whether or not you need an exercise stress test. A stress test will detect any inappropriate reaction to exercise including a sudden change in blood pressure, angina or chest pain, arrhythmias due to exertion, and other problems.

I usually allow my thirty-five- to forty-five-year-old women to forego the stress test if they are healthy and do not have any risk factors (such as high blood pressure, diabetes, or elevated cholesterol) that could possibly be irritated by exercise. All patients over forty-five should be given a stress test. Based on the results, the physician can tailor an exercise program to the individual patient.

For previously sedentary patients, I usually prescribe a simple, easy-to-follow walking program that they can do on their own. I particularly encourage women to walk because no special equipment is required. Walking also helps tone up muscles in the legs, hips, and trouble spots where there is often the highest concentration of fat in the female body. My goal is to get everyone to walk two miles a day, at a brisk pace—roughly 3–4 mph—a minimum of three days a week. Some women will eventually achieve the goal; others will stop at a lesser level. Some women may prefer to walk a mile or two a day over five days, and that's okay too.

Week 1: Try walking a half a mile at a time (roughly 10 city blocks total, or 5 blocks each way). If you don't live in a city, try the local school track or first log the distance in your car around the neighborhood. Each walk should take about 25 minutes. (This is not a race. Go slower if you have to.) Try to walk at least three times a week, preferably five. Stick to areas where there is pretty scenery or there are interesting things to look at to help fight boredom. Avoid walking in isolated areas by yourself. Do not go out at night alone. If you get tired or out of breath, sit down and rest and then continue your walk. *If you experience any dizziness, pain, or unusual symptoms, discontinue your walk and call your doctor.*

Week 2: If you feel that you can, try increasing the walk to 15 blocks, or 7.5 blocks each way. If you don't want to do it all at once, add an extra block every day until you reach 15. The walk should take between 25 and 30 minutes, but go slower if you have to.

Week 3: You're up to a mile. Try for 10 blocks each way. Try to keep it between 25 and 30 minutes, but don't push it. If you need to sit down and rest, do it.

Week 4: Add 5 more blocks each way to 15 blocks. See if you can do it within 25 to 30 minutes.

Week 5: Add 5 more blocks each way to 20 blocks. You are now walking two miles. Try to keep within 30 to 35 minutes if you can.

Taking Your Target Heart Rate

If you're happy with your walking program the way it is, don't bother making any changes. However, if you're motivated to do more, you can make sure that you are achieving maximum cardiovascular benefit from your walking regime by learning how to take your target heart rate. The target heart rate is based on the patient's age, health, state of fitness, and other factors. If you take a stress test, your target heart rate would be derived from the maximum heart rate achieved at peak exertion. For example, if your heartbeat went up to 180 beats per minute during the stress test, your target heart rate would be between 70 percent and 85 percent of that number. However, if you were in poor physical condition, your target heart rate might even be lower to start, but would gradually increase as you became more fit. If you haven't had a stress test, you can figure out your target heart rate yourself by using the following formula:

1. Subtract your age from 220 to determine your maximum heart rate. For example, based on this formula, if you're forty years old, your maximum heart rate would be 180.
2. Since you shouldn't push yourself to your outermost limit, your target heart rate would then be anywhere from 70 percent to 85 percent of that number, depending on your level of fitness (126–153).
3. To measure your heart rate, simply put your finger on your wrist or carotid artery (located on the left side of your neck) to feel your pulse. Measure the number of throbs you feel per ten-second interval. Then multiply that number by 6.

When you start your walk, go at a slow, comfortable pace. Gradually pick up your speed. Once you achieve your target heart rate, continue walking at that pace for about 20 minutes. Then slowly wind down until your heart rate has returned to normal—around 72 beats per minute. If you feel sick, dizzy, or experience any unusual symptoms, slow down gradually and call your doctor.

COMMONSENSE EXERCISE

Despite the adage "no pain, no gain," exercise should never hurt. Even if you're working hard, you should always feel comfortable. The rule of thumb is that you should never exercise beyond the point at which you are able to carry on a conversation. In fact, there's some evidence to suggest that overexerting yourself may actually be counterproductive.

When you exercise, your body utilizes more oxygen. Ideally, you should consume enough oxygen to meet the increased need—this is called steady state. When you achieve steady state, your body begins to break down fat, which burns up calories. At steady state, you should be able to exercise comfortably for 20 or 30 minutes. But if you exercise beyond your ability to consume oxygen, you will be working in oxygen debt. In this condition, you begin to burn up predominantly carbohydrate calories, leaving your fat stores intact, which doesn't help to eliminate excess pounds. To make matters worse, without enough oxygen, you will not be able to sustain the exercise for any significant amount of time. In other words, you'll burn out.

WHAT IF WALKING IS NOT FOR YOU?

Although walking is terrific for most people, there are some people who simply don't like it. For some women, swimming, tennis, or a dance class are a lot more palatable than walking.

Some women may be motivated enough to exercise on their own, but others may need the camaraderie of a class at a gym or health club, or the discipline offered by a personal exercise trainer. But before you agree to put your body in somebody else's hands, let me tell about my experience.

A few years ago, I felt that I needed to get more exercise. I knew that if I tried to do it alone I would never stick with it, but because of my hectic schedule I couldn't commit to a class. So I decided to hire a personal trainer, highly recommended by a close friend, who agreed to come to my home early in the morning. I paid in advance for ten sessions, but unfortunately never made it through my first. Although I had advised the trainer that I had an injured disk in my neck, she insisted that I "work through" any discomfort I was feeling. I made the mistake of assuming that this woman knew what she was doing. Despite the twinges and stabbing pain, I kept going until finally I realized that this was insanity.

I fired the trainer, but it was too late. That hour of exercise cost me six weeks in a neck brace and hours of discomfort. This experience will not have been in vain if I can pass this advice onto other women. Just because someone calls herself an exercise trainer doesn't mean she knows the first thing about either exercise or training. In fact, anyone can call herself an exercise trainer or teacher: There is no regulatory agency that oversees this profession. So when it comes to choosing an exercise instructor—either your own personal trainer or one at a health club—the name of the game is consumer beware. Many clubs offer a dazzling array of exercise equipment and machinery, Olympic-size swimming pools, and classes in everything from martial arts to aerobics. But don't be impressed by glitz—keep in mind that a club is only as good as the people who are working there.

After my bad experience, I checked with the American College of Sports Medicine, a professional organization that accredits exercise personnel and facilities, to see what advice they would have about finding a good sports facility or locating a qualified exercise trainer or teacher. According to Bill Gillespie, Ph.D., an exercise physiologist who is on the group's certification committee, health consumers have to do their homework. First, if you're thinking of joining a health club or gym, find out if the facility is accredited by the American College of Sports Medicine. The seal of approval from this group means that the facility conforms to certain standards and the personnel are well trained. However, Gillespie admits that many health facilities have not even applied for certification, which doesn't necessarily mean that the facility is bad. In this case, the consumer must do additional checking.

For example, make sure that the exercise teachers have a minimum of a B.A. degree from an accredited institution in either physical education, exercise physiology, or health and fitness. People with this kind of training generally know how to help others work out safely and effectively. In some of the more reputable clubs, the managers are required to have a master's degree. If the teachers lack the proper educational credentials, Gillespie advises people to walk out.

He also cautions consumers to be aware of clubs that have their own "quickie" training programs: Six weeks in a health club observing other members of the staff does not provide enough knowledge or experience to bestow the title of exercise trainer. Often these clubs hire people who look good in shorts or a leotard rather than those who are truly qualified. Just because someone knows how to take care of her own body doesn't mean she knows how to take care of yours. This same advice applies if you are hiring a personal trainer: Make sure she has both the credentials and the experience to do the job.

Before beginning an exercise program, tell your teacher or trainer about any orthopedic or other health problems that you may have. A good teacher will be careful not to allow you to strain or hurt yourself in any way. Most clubs or trainers will want a letter from your physician certifying that you are in good health.

You should always stop exercising at the first sign of trouble. Be sure to call your doctor if you experience any unusual symptoms including the following:

1. Shortness of breath
2. Chest pain
3. Dizziness
4. Heart palpitations
5. Pain anywhere in your body

FOR WOMEN WITH HEART DISEASE

Up until now, I've talked about exercise as a way to control the risk factors that can lead to heart disease. But exercise also has an important role in the rehabilitative process that begins after a heart attack or upon receiving a diagnosis of CAD.

The goal of a rehabilitation program is to improve cardiac function and to

RESOURCES: For information on health clubs see page 235.

lower the resting heart rate. If the patient has CAD but has not had a heart attack, exercise may help eliminate some of the risk factors that could lead to a myocardial infarction. If the patient has already had a heart attack, an exercise program will not only tone up the remaining heart muscle that is still working but may actually increase her life span.

According to one recent study of men after a heart attack (sorry, women were not included), those who exercised four hours a week had a lower death rate after two years than those who remained sedentary. Although exercise did not reduce their rate of recurrence for heart attack, it did increase longevity. It probably also improved their quality of life. Exercise not only builds up muscle but often helps to build up self-esteem. After a heart attack people often feel betrayed by their bodies. They see themselves embarking on a downward cycle that inevitably leads to disability and then death. But when these people start exercising, they begin to see wonderful changes in their bodies. Their muscles firm up, they slim down, and they look more fit. Ironically, many women actually feel much better about themselves during the post–heart attack period than they ever did before.

After a heart attack, an exercise rehabilitation plan is usually divided into four phases:

1. *Phase 1:* The early stages of physical fitness begin in the hospital where the patient is encouraged to engage in very low levels of activity usually involving self-care: combing her hair, brushing her teeth, and walking to the bathroom. Before she leaves the hospital, she will be asked to take a "mini" stress test in which her heart rate is allowed to rise to about 120 and no further. Based on the results of the stress test, her doctor will design a posthospital exercise routine.

2. *Phase 2:* This next critical stage is a very limited personalized exercise regimen that the patient does at home. It may not include anything more taxing than slow walking and mild calisthenics done in a rest position. Patients are taught a new way of measuring activity in units of energy called mets. One met is equal to the amount of oxygen needed to maintain your body while sitting down—approximately 3.5 milliliters of oxygen per body weight per minute. All activity can be measured in terms of mets. For example, it takes 3 mets to rake leaves, 5 to play a game of tennis (singles), and 9 to jog at the rate of 5 mph. The goal is to get the patient up to performing 3 to 5 mets of activity without fatigue or other symptoms. In doing so, the goal is to give the patient an awareness of how she is using her body and to alleviate fears of overexertion. Six weeks after achieving this goal (usually around four months post–heart attack) the patient should have another exercise stress test, this time limited only by the occurrence of symptoms. When this test is evaluated, the patient

can then be trained further to achieve even better function of the heart and lungs.

3. *Phase 3:* Patients who are mending well are often referred to a cardiac rehabilitation center, an exercise facility specially designed for people with cardiac problems. Some of these cardiac fitness centers are affiliated with hospitals; others are run independently. Whether or not the center is connected to a medical facility, the program should be overseen by a cardiologist. In a well-run center, a nurse should be on site at all times. The exercise instructors should have a B.A. in physical fitness or another related field as well as additional training in cardiac rehabilitation.

Ideally, the facility and the staff should be certified by the American College of Sports Medicine. Certification from this group is your assurance that the exercise leaders or trainers are qualified to work with cardiac patients, and can tailor their approach based on the individual patient. For example, patients who are taking certain medications may react differently to exercise. It is often up to the trainer to distinguish between "normal" irregularities due to the drug or more ominous ones due to other problems. Therefore, it's critical for the exercise trainer to understand the patient's medical history and general physical state. A good exercise program should begin very gradually under the supervision of qualified personnel. Over time, the cardiac patient can gradually increase her exercise program as she builds up her tolerance.

4. *Phase 4:* Six months later, the patient may be able to leave the protective care of the cardiac center and begin to exercise on her own. Many patients, however, prefer to remain affiliated with their program, enjoying both the camaraderie of working with other people and the security of close supervision.

If you have a cardiac problem, you must talk to your doctor before embarking on an exercise program. Although most cardiac patients can exercise safely, there are some people who should not, at least until their condition is stabilized and their doctors have given their approval. They include:

1. Women with unstable angina, that is, angina that is increasing in frequency or intensity although the work remains the same
2. Women who have just had an acute heart attack
3. Women with blood pressure greater than 200/110
4. Women with any arrhythmia that could compromise cardiac function
5. Women with severe narrowing or stenosis of the aorta
6. Women with inflammation of the heart muscle
7. Women with any cardiac problem that poses a risk to her health

Chapter 19

A WOMAN'S DIET
AND HEART DISEASE

A woman's diet—both what and how much she eats—can have a profound effect on her risk of developing CAD. Consider the following:

- A woman who eats a diet high in saturated fat and cholesterol is more likely to have cholesterol levels of more than 240 mg/dl, high levels of LDL (the "bad" cholesterol), and low levels of HDL (the "good" cholesterol).
- About 20 percent of the adult population is obese—that is, 20 percent to 30 percent above normal body weight. Obesity appears to be a serious risk factor for heart attack in women. According to a recent study, 70 percent of all heart attacks in obese women and 40 percent in women overall are related to excess weight. Women who are obese are also more likely to have high blood pressure and triglyceride blood levels higher than 190 mg/dl, thus increasing their risk of developing CAD and stroke. They are also are more likely to develop diabetes, an inability to metabolize blood sugar. Diabetes greatly increases a woman's risk of heart attack.
- Women who are chronic "weight cyclers"—that is, they lose and gain weight rapidly—are at greater risk of having a heart attack than women who maintain a stable weight.

Eating the right food and maintaining an appropriate weight for your age, frame, and body build can be your best defense against CAD. In many ways, dieting is counterproductive: 90 percent of all people who begin a diet regime eventually quit, usually out of boredom and frustration. It's important for everyone to have a basic understanding of heart-healthy nutrition. Once you understand the rules, it's very simple to incorporate them into your life without turning it upside down.

WATCH YOUR FAT INTAKE

Although eating excess amounts of the wrong kind of fat can promote heart disease, fat is a necessary part of life. A woman's body is composed of approximately 25 percent to 35 percent fatty tissue—about 10 percent more than a man's body. She needs the extra fat to sustain her through pregnancy and lactation, which are both times of increased energy demand.

Body fat also serves several other vital functions: It provides a reserve of energy during times of famine or diet; it carries the fat-soluble vitamins A, D, E, and K throughout the body; it protects and insulates body organs; it is essential in the manufacture of certain hormones including estrogen. In fact, if a woman's level of body fat drops below 25 percent, she may suffer from amenorrhea—that is, she will stop menstruating. This often happens to female athletes who have a greater proportion of muscle-to-fat than normal, and to anorexic women who are on very low-calorie diets of 800 calories or less over a prolonged period.

Fat is also an excellent source of energy. Calories are the way we measure the energy provided by fat and the two other basic nutrients: protein and carbohydrate.

· It takes 3,500 extra calories to create 1 pound of body fat.
· One gram of fat equals 9 calories.
· One gram of protein or carbohydrate equals 4 calories

Some foods contain just one type of nutrient; others are a combination of two or three. Fatty cuts of meat, whole milk dairy products, salad dressings, and baked goods are just some examples of the commonly consumed foods that are laden with fat calories. But the body has the capacity to convert any excess energy (calories) intake into fat—in other words, you don't have to eat fat to store fat. Routinely eating more calories than you expend will result in being overweight.

There are three different forms of dietary fat: saturated fats, polyunsaturated fats, and monounsaturated fats. As a rule, the more saturated the fat, the more solid it is at room temperature, and the more unsaturated the fat, the more liquid it is at room temperature.

According to the American Heart Association, people should eat no more than 30 percent of their daily calories in the form of any kind of fat and no more than 300 mg of cholesterol per day. If you consider that the average woman consumes 1,800 calories daily, you should eat no more than 540 calories in the form of any fat.

Saturated Fats

WHAT ARE THEY?

These fats are primarily found in food of animal origin including fatty cuts of beef, lamb, butter, and to a lesser extent, chicken and fish. Although they are derived from plants, coconut oil and palm kernel oil are also high in saturated fats. Some foods that are high in saturated fats are also high in cholesterol, such as eggs (one egg contains 273 mg of cholesterol) and liver (3 ounces of cooked liver contains 410 mg).

However, saturated fats from plant sources, such as coconut oil and peanut butter, have no cholesterol. Nevertheless, these foods do not get a clean bill of health. Saturated fat from any source—animal or vegetable—may stimulate the body to increase its production of cholesterol, especially LDL, or the so-called "bad" cholesterol. Therefore, keep in mind that many foods that are promoted as cholesterol-free such as peanut butter and baked goods containing palm or coconut oils still contain saturated fat that may directly raise blood cholesterol. These foods should be eaten in moderation.

DAILY ALLOWANCE.

According to the dietary guidelines of the American Heart Association, people should not consume more than 10 percent of their total calories in the form of saturated fat. This means eating no more than 3 to 4 ounces of the leanest cuts of meat, skinless chicken, or fish (poached, broiled, or baked) per serving no more than twice a day. It also means switching to low-fat or no-fat dairy products. People with high cholesterol levels may need to reduce their daily intake of saturated fat to as little as 7 percent or less of their daily calories. As of this writing, food manufacturers are not required to list the total percentage of calories derived from saturated fat on their product labels. Therefore, it is up to the consumer to be aware of which products are high in saturated fat.

Polyunsaturated Fats

WHAT ARE THEY?

These fats are found mainly in vegetable oils or margarines made from vegetable sources. Good sources include safflower, soybean, corn, cotton seed, sesame, and sunflower oils. (These oils also have small amounts of saturated and monounsaturated fats.) Polyunsaturated oils contain linoleic acid, a critical ingredient in the formation of cells and the functioning of the nervous system. Since the body cannot produce linoleic acid on its own, it must derive this important building block from food. Although highly unsaturated fats have been shown to reduce blood cholesterol levels, they are also high in calories. In addition, diets high in polyunsaturated fats have been linked to breast and rectal cancers and the formation of gallstones. Too many dietary polyunsaturates may also inhibit the formation of white blood cells, which is important for immune function.

Not all polyunsaturated oils are as beneficial as others. Some polyunsaturated oils and all margarines undergo a process called hydrogenation to increase their shelf life and make them useful for baking. This process increases their degree of saturation, thus decreasing their ability to cut cholesterol, but they are still nutritionally better than butter or lard. The more hydrogenated the margarine, the harder and more saturated it becomes. Therefore, try to buy only partially hydrogenated soft margarine that is sold in tubs. Make sure the primary ingredient—the first one listed on the label—is a highly polyunsaturated oil such as corn or safflower. For cooking, stick to oils that are not hydrogenated.

DAILY ALLOWANCE.

Total intake of polyunsaturated fats should not exceed 10 percent of daily calories. Each teaspoon of any kind of fat contains 45 calories. However, since hidden sources of fat are found in so much of the food we eat, I recommend that you not add more than 2 to 3 teaspoons of polyunsaturated fat to your food daily. (Keep in mind that 1 pat of margarine equals 1 teaspoon fat). Since condiments such as salad dressing and mayonnaise are basically oil (unless they are the no-oil variety), use them very sparingly. Another form of polyunsaturated fats are omega-3 fatty acids.

Omega-3 Fatty Acids

WHAT ARE THEY?

Certain types of foods—mostly fish—are rich in a type of polyunsaturated fat known as omega-3 fatty acids. Omega-3 fatty acids not only lower blood cholesterol but unlike vegetable oils they also reduce blood triglyceride levels, which is especially important for women. Omega-3s also inhibit the clotting action of blood, thus reducing the risk of developing a clot that could break off and block an artery to the heart or brain.

The best sources of omega-3 are white tuna, salmon, mackerel, herring, lake trout, and to a lesser extent, cod, flounder, and halibut. Keep in mind that the positive effects of fish can be reduced if you prepare it in a heart-unhealthy manner, such as frying it in a highly saturated fat or smothering it in butter or a mayonnaise sauce. The best way to prepare fish is to bake, broil, poach, or steam it, using as little fat as possible. Walnuts and butternuts are also good sources of omega-3, but ounce for ounce they are higher in calories than fish.

In some parts of the United States, certain species of fish have been tainted due to water pollution and should not be eaten. If you're unsure about which varieties may be affected in your area, call your local health department or regional office of the Environmental Protection Agency.

DAILY ALLOWANCE.

Every woman should eat 1 ounce of fresh fish daily or two fish meals a week (3 to 4-ounce servings). There is no evidence yet that fish oil tablets sold in drug and health food stores provide the same benefits as eating the real thing.

Monounsaturated Fats

WHAT ARE THEY?

Oleic acid is the prime ingredient in this group of fats found in abundance in several common cooking oils, including olive oil, rapeseed (canola oil), and some forms of sunflower seed and safflower oil. Until recently it was believed that these types of fats had a neutral effect on cholesterol; that is, they neither raised it nor lowered it. But we know now that this isn't true. According to the latest findings, fats in olive oil not only lower cholesterol like polyunsaturated oils but manage to do so without lowering the beneficial HDL. A study in Italy showed that people who ate diets rich in olive oil had the lowest levels of blood cholesterol, blood pressure, and blood glucose.

DAILY ALLOWANCE.

Although researchers were unsure why monounsaturated fats had such a beneficial effect, they were certain of one thing: Americans should eat more monounsaturated fats and less saturated fats. In fact, some researchers now recommend increasing intake of monounsaturates to 10 percent to 15 percent of our daily calories, and in turn, reducing our intake of saturated and polyunsaturated fats. Routinely sprinkling 2 to 3 teaspoons of olive oil on your salad or vegetables and using a monounsaturated cooking oil such as rapeseed or canola should do the trick.

For most of us, restricting our fat intake to 30 percent will require some modest changes in diet. In fact, the average American eats a diet that is between 40 percent and 50 percent fat, and much of it is in the form of saturated fat. Compared to other cuisines in the world, the American diet is low in complex carbohydrates (fruits, vegetables, and grains) and high in protein, especially meat, which is high in calories and saturated fat.

I asked nutrition counselor Marianne Sciberras, M.S., R.D., to whom I often refer patients, to devise an easy-to-follow daily diet plan for women that would meet all the necessary requirements without being too confining. If you follow these guidelines, you will be eating both wisely and well.

DAILY RECOMMENDED SERVINGS FOR WOMEN EIGHTEEN AND OLDER

	Women 18–24	Women 25+	Women Pregnant/ Nursing	Teens Pregnant/ Nursing
Dairy	4	2	4	5
Protein	2	2	2	2
Fruits	2–4	2–4	2–4	2–4
Vegetables	3–5	3–5	3–5	3–5
Grains	6	6	6	6

DAIRY:

Major source of calcium, protein, and riboflavin

RECOMMENDED SERVING:

1 cup skim milk (1% or ½% fat)
   or
1 cup low-fat yogurt
1½ slices low-fat cheese
½ cup ice milk or frozen yogurt

PROTEIN:

Major source of iron

RECOMMENDED SERVING:

3 oz cooked lean beef, fish, or poultry without skin

PROTEIN EQUIVALENTS FOR 2 OZ MEAT:

4 tbsp peanut butter
2 eggs, preferably 1 yolk with two whites, or ¼ cup of substitute
1 cup dried beans: navy, black, or pinto
½ cup cottage cheese (if cottage cheese is used as a meat substitute do not also count it as a dairy)

FRUITS OR VEGETABLES:

Major source of fiber, vitamins (especially A & C) and minerals

RECOMMENDED SERVINGS:

　　$^1\!/_2$ cup cooked or canned fruit or vegetables
　　1 cup raw vegetables
　　1 medium-size orange, apple, pear, banana, plum (if small, allow two)
　　$^1\!/_4$ cup dried fruit or $^1\!/_2$ cup berries
　　$^1\!/_2$ grapefruit or $^3\!/_4$ cup juice

GRAINS:

Major source of fiber, B vitamins, iron (if enriched), niacin, and thiamin; whole-grain, fortified, and/or enriched products are recommended

RECOMMENDED SERVINGS:

　　1 slice bread, $^1\!/_2$ bagel, medium-size roll,
　　　3–4 small crackers or 2 large crackers
　　$^3\!/_4$ cup or 1 oz dry cereal or $^1\!/_2$ cup cooked cereal
　　$^1\!/_2$ cup cooked pasta, rice, bulgar, barley, or cornmeal

Adapted from guidelines issued by the National Dairy Council.

HEART-HEALTHY FOOD TIPS

Trim the Meat

Any meat portion—whether it is beef, fish, or fowl—should be no more than 3 to 4 ounces per serving.

- If you eat red meat, buy beef that is rated "select" because it is the leanest. Stick to cuts that are naturally low in fat, such as flank steak, round steak, trimmed tenderloin, sirloin-tip steak, and center-cut ham. If you buy chopped meat, have your butcher grind an extra lean variety made from the above cuts. Store-bought chopped meat can be well over 50 percent fat.
- Avoid hot dogs, luncheon meats, and other processed meats because they are high in processed fats and sodium. If you must eat processed meat, look for brands that are over 95 percent fat-free.

- Eat more fatty fish, such as white tuna, mackerel, and salmon, which is an excellent source of omega-3.
- Skinless, white-meat chicken has about half the fat of red meat, and is lower in calories.
- All meats—beef, poultry, and fowl—should be prepared with as little fat as possible.

Get Enough Iron

Despite the saturated fat, red meat is an important source of iron, which is essential for menstruating women. Although iron is also found in dried white beans, enriched breads and cereals, and other plant foods, heme, or iron from animal sources, is better utilized by the body. Iron is best absorbed with a vitamin C source, such as orange juice or broccoli. Coffee, tea, and alcohol inhibit iron absorption and should be used in moderation.

Women Need More Calcium

Most dairy products are a good source of dietary calcium, which is necessary to prevent osteoporosis, or thinning of the bones. Calcium also plays a critical role in the functioning of the heart and other muscles. According to the surgeon general's report on nutrition and health, most American women do not get the full recommended daily allowance (RDA) of calcium. Women between nineteen and twenty-four need 1,200 milligrams of calcium daily. Women twenty-five and older need 800 milligrams. By simply consuming between two and four dairy foods daily, along with a well-balanced diet, you can be certain that you are getting enough of this vital element. Since milk products can be rich in saturated fat, use low-fat products only.

The calcium from milk is better absorbed if it's taken along with a well-balanced meal than if it's consumed by itself between meals. If a diet is too high in protein or salt, calcium will be excreted by the bones. If you can't eat milk products due to a lactose intolerance, try using lactose-free dairy products. Good nondairy sources of calcium include:

½ cup fresh cooked spinach	122 mg
1 tbsp Blackstrap molasses	137 mg
½ cup turnip greens	99 mg

Increase Fiber

Grains, fruits, and vegetables are all excellent sources of dietary fiber. Fiber is a type of complex carbohydrate that is a component of many of these nutritious foods. Although fiber is indigestible and provides no nutrients or calories, it plays a critical role in our bodies. There are two types of fiber: soluble and insoluble. Insoluble fiber, typically found in foods such as celery, wheat bran, kidney beans, and pinto beans, helps prevent constipation by speeding up the movement of food through the intestine. Many studies suggest that a diet high in insoluble fiber can help prevent cancer of the colon, diverticulosis, and other digestive disorders.

Soluble fiber, found in oat bran, rice bran, apples, broccoli, citrus fruits, and root vegetables, slows down the movement of food through the intestine. Studies have shown that soluble fiber also lowers total blood cholesterol, which reduces the risk of CAD. Although we're not exactly sure why soluble fiber has such a beneficial effect on cholesterol, researchers suspect that it works in a roundabout way. Soluble fiber binds with bile in the intestine and is excreted in the feces. The liver compensates for the loss of bile by producing more bile salts, of which cholesterol is a necessary ingredient, thus lowering the level of this fat in the blood. Combined with a low-fat diet, an adequate amount of fiber can lower blood triglyceride levels.

On average, Americans eat only half the amount of fiber that experts now believe is necessary for a healthy diet. A well-rounded diet should include between 20 and 40 grams of fiber—if possible, half soluble, half insoluble. Don't gorge yourself on either kind of fiber. Too much fiber can cause diarrhea and an upset stomach, as well as interfere with the absorption of essential dietary minerals such as calcium and iron. If your diet has been low in fiber, gradually increase your consumption over several weeks until your body has adjusted to the change.

Cut Down on Salt

Most of us eat a lot more salt than our bodies need to run efficiently—in fact, a mere 500 milligrams is all we really need. Daily intake of sodium should be limited to 2,400 milligrams per day, or 1,000 milligrams for every 1,000 calories. This may sound like a lot of sodium, but consider the sodium contents in the following:

Fast-food deluxe hamburger	1,200 mg
1 tbsp soy sauce	800 mg
1 tbsp salad dressing	80–250 mg
½ cup canned vegetables or beans	400 mg

Seventy-five percent of all dietary sodium comes from processed foods—luncheon meats, sausage, condiments, commerical tomato sauces, vegetables, and juices are especially high in sodium. To cut down on salt, you need to restrict severely the amount of processed food in your diet, or switch to the low-salt or no-salt variety.

Don't use a commercial salt substitute unless it has been approved by your doctor. Many of these products contain potassium, which may not be safe for people with kidney disorders or other medical problems.

Eat Less But More Often

We live in a culture where three meals a day is the norm, but ideally people should eat six smaller meals a day, or three moderate meals and two healthy but small snacks. Eating smaller amounts more frequently helps activate your metabolism and keeps it operating at peak efficiency. Here's an added bonus: Studies show that smaller meals throughout the day lower cholesterol and blood sugar and raise the beneficial HDL in women as well as men.

HOW CAN EATING HABITS BE CHANGED?

When I encounter a patient who needs to make changes in her diet because of health problems, such as high cholesterol or high triglycerides, I usually refer her to a dietitian for counseling. Although it is possible to change your eating habits on your own, I feel it is helpful to have the moral support and knowledge provided by a trained counselor. It is essential to work with a trained nutritional counselor if you are obese, or have any other dietary problem such as diabetes, or an eating disorder such as anorexia. Be sure to choose a counselor who is a registered dietitian (R.D.), which means that she is accredited by The American Dietetic Association, or ADA.

A good nutrition counselor will learn a lot about the patient before making any recommendations. First, she will discuss the patient with the referring doctor, reviewing the patient's medical problems and reasons for referral. The nutrition counselor and the doctor will jointly set goals for the patient, and formulate a strategy to help the patient succeed. Then the counselor will take her own careful medical history to determine if the patient is at risk for any particular problems.

The next step is to ask the patient to keep a careful food diary for at least a week—a log of everything she has eaten including snacks—to get a sense of her caloric intake and eating habits. The diary also includes such details as the time you ate and the place, what you were doing, how long it took, and other relevant facts. From the diary, the counselor will also get an idea of the patient's likes and dislikes, as well as any patterns that need changing. Based on the patient's weight, age, activity level, medical history, and food preferences, the counselor will devise an eating plan specifically tailored for that patient.

The counselor should also take the patient's lifestyle into account, accommodating coffee breaks, cocktail hours, and dining in fast-food restaurants. A good nutrition counselor knows that the best eating plans are the ones that allow the patient to make small, incremental changes that are simple and easy to follow. A rigid, difficult diet may look great on paper, but it is useless if it cannot be easily incorporated into the patient's everyday life.

If the patient has to lose weight, the goal should be for no more than 1 to 2 pounds per week for as long as it takes. If you are experiencing a period of emotional turbulence—for example, you're going through a divorce or have recently lost your job—it may not be the right time to attempt to lose weight. A weight-loss program requires energy and optimism. It's better to wait until things calm down than to try and fail.

Often, tremendous gains can be achieved by making modest changes in a patient's eating style. To prove my point, I have included two food diaries kept by two women whom I referred to Marianne for counseling. First, you will see the patient's food log, which is followed by recommended changes.

CASE HISTORY 1:
SHELLEY B.

AGE: 55
HEIGHT: 5'4"
WEIGHT: 138 lb
CHOLESTEROL: 288 (high)
HDL: 40 (too low)
TRIGLYCERIDES: 160 (normal)
BLOOD PRESSURE: 140/95 (high)

Goals

Shelley's mother had a heart attack in her fifties, and Shelley wants to prevent that from happening to her. She is highly motivated and concerned about her health, but believes that she is eating a well-balanced diet and feels that she can't do much better than she is doing now. Fortunately, her triglycerides are normal, but her cholesterol is high and her HDL-to-total-cholesterol ratio is below 6:1, which is considered poor. Combined with high blood pressure, this puts Shelley at greater risk of heart attack and stroke. For her petite frame, her weight is more than 10 pounds above the acceptable limit based on the Metropolitan Life tables. Shelley has put on a few pounds recently and would like to take them off. To reduce her risk factors, Shelley must reduce her cholesterol level and lower her blood pressure. Weight reduction will very likely help her to achieve these goals.

Shelley's Food Diary (A Typical Day)

BREAKFAST AT HOME

6 oz orange juice
³/₄ cup corn flakes
8 oz 2% low-fat milk
2 tsp sugar

LUNCH BROUGHT FROM HOME

2 slices low-calorie bread
1½ oz ham luncheon meat
1½ tsp regular mayonnaise
coffee with cream
1 apple, peeled

DINNER AT HOME

8 oz broiled steak
1 cup cooked broccoli
1 tsp butter
1 baked potato
1 tbsp sour cream and chives
1 banana
8 oz soda water with twist lemon
4 medium chocolate chip cookies
1 scoop premium vanilla fudge ice cream

Diagnosis and Prescription

Shelley also reported that although her typical workday is busy, she rarely gets much exercise. She drives to work, takes an elevator to her fourth-floor office, occasionally sunbathes in the plaza outside her office building at lunch, and takes her dog on short walks of about a block or so.

Although Shelley's 24-hour recall of her diet shows that it is fairly well balanced, there is still considerable room for improvement. For one thing, she needs to reduce her intake of meat. Eight ounces in one sitting is too much. With both high cholesterol and high blood pressure, she also needs to restrict her intake of hidden fat and sodium. She should try to eliminate processed foods, such as luncheon meat, from her diet or to use the new low-sodium, low-fat varieties.

Shelley also needs to eat more fiber-rich foods. Fiber not only will help her feel fuller and prevent overeating, but by replacing higher fat and salty foods, it can also help reduce blood pressure. Shelley's diet is also lacking adequate food from the milk group. She is short the two minimum servings a day needed for women twenty-five and older and is not meeting her RDAs for calcium. Calcium is not only necessary to prevent osteoporosis but it also helps regulate blood pressure. Although ice cream provides some calcium (but not as much as low-fat milk), the premium brand that Shelley likes is extremely high in calories (280 calories per scoop or 4-ounce serving) and fat (14 grams). If she craves something chocolate and cold at the end of her dinner, she should switch to low-fat frozen chocolate yogurt at about 130 calories per serving and only 3 grams of fat.

It is very important for Shelley to incorporate some forms of activity into her very sedentary lifestyle. She could try walking her dog for 20 to 30 minutes a day, instead of just around the block. As you will see, none of our recommendations are too difficult to follow, but even minor changes in eating habits and lifestyle can reap dramatic improvements.

Recommended Diet

BREAKFAST

1 medium orange	Whole fruit is a better source of fiber than juice.
¾ cup grapenut flakes or raisin bran	These cereals are much lower in sodium than most ready-to-eat or instant cereals.
8 oz skim milk in cereal	
8 oz coffee with 2% low-fat milk	This milk is appreciably lower in fat than cream, but it still has the desired effect on the coffee, whereas the substitution of skim milk in coffee often sends dieters racing back for cream.
2 tsp sugar	Only 32 calories and good for the soul.

LUNCH BROUGHT FROM HOME

2 slices cracked wheat or oatmeal bread	It's higher in fiber and more satisfying than diet white bread.
1½ oz sliced fresh turkey breast	It's lower in calories and sodium than processed luncheon meat and just as satisfying.
1½ tsp diet mayonnaise	It's lower in fat than the regular stuff and these days many brands actually taste good!
1 apple with skin on	Skin provides fiber and added nutrition since vitamins and minerals are closer to the surface of the fruit.

DINNER

3–4 oz broiled steak trimmed of all visible fat

1 cup cooked broccoli sautéed in 1 tbsp olive oil and chopped garlic

Olive oil helps cut cholesterol without cutting HDL.

1 baked potato with skin

1 tbsp plain nonfat yogurt and chives

Non-fat yogurt is lower in fat, calories, and sodium than sour cream. Mixed with chives, it's hard to distinguish from sour cream.

no-salt seltzer and twist of lemon or lime

1 banana or 12 grapes

EVENING SNACK

4 ginger snaps plus 8 oz skim milk

At 3 grams of fat per serving, ginger snaps are much lower in fat than chocolate chip cookies.

or

4 oz low-fat chocolate frozen yogurt mixed with 4 oz milk

A delicious low-calorie "milkshake."

Six Months Later

Shelley's cholesterol was down to 245, and her blood pressure was down to 130/80. Her HDL rose slightly to 45, but the HDL-to-total-cholesterol ratio has improved. Not only does she feel better but without officially dieting she has managed to shed 5 pounds, undoubtedly due to her moderately increased activity level and her better eating habits. Shelley is now eating a truly well-balanced diet that is lower in calories, fat, and salt, and higher in fiber and calcium.

CASE HISTORY 2:
LUCY R.

AGE: 42
HEIGHT: 5'5"
WEIGHT: 165 lb
CHOLESTEROL: 275 (high)
HDL: 35 (poor)
TRIGLYCERIDES: 355 (high)
BLOOD PRESSURE: 140/90 (borderline high)

Goals

Based on her medium frame, Lucy is 25 pounds overweight; her cholesterol is high, with the HDL-to-cholesterol ratio higher than 6:1; and her triglycerides are considerably above the normal upper limit of 190. Her blood pressure is borderline high, which is worrisome, considering her other vital statistics.

Lucy is under a great deal of pressure at work and she says she eats when she's nervous. She strongly resists the concept of dieting and doesn't want to give up her favorite foods, which include chocolate and soda. She says she hates all forms of exercise, except she used to like swimming when she was in college.

To reduce her risk factors for CAD, Lucy must lose some weight, and reduce her triglycerides and cholesterol.

Lucy's Food Diary (A Typical Day)

BREAKFAST AT COFFEE SHOP

4 strips bacon and 2 eggs on a buttered roll
tea with half-and-half (mixture of milk and cream)
2 tsp sugar

MIDMORNING SNACK

2-oz package M&Ms
2 brownies
8 oz cola

LUNCH AT RESTAURANT

1 slice pizza
8 oz cola

SNACK

2 brownies
8 oz cola

DINNER AT HOME

2 beef hot dogs (average 13 grams fat)
2 buns
2 tbsp mustard
2 beers
small bag potato chips (1½ oz)
½ cup canned peaches

EVENING SNACK

2-oz. pack M&Ms
2 beers
1½ oz potato chips

Diagnosis and Prescription

Lucy's 24-hour record shows that her diet is high in fat, sugar, and sodium and low in fiber and calcium. Her eating style, however, is not that unusual for someone who eats for reasons other than hunger or who doesn't understand the basics of good nutrition. She also consumes too much alcohol, which is very high in calories. At 7 calories per gram, alcohol is nearly as caloric as fat. Since pouring a drink or two at night to unwind had become second nature to her, Lucy herself was surprised by how much she had been drinking. Since she has made it clear that she is not willing to make any major changes in her eating or lifestyle, all we could do was show her how she could modify her current diet to make a few healthful improvements.

Although Lucy hates to exercise, she can learn to incorporate some physical activity into her life the easy way. It doesn't have to be in the form of exercise as we know it. Walking, dancing, or even window shopping is a big improvement over sitting still. Since she doesn't mind swimming, it would be terrific if she could find a place to swim at least once a week. In addition, if she is to reduce her triglycerides to a safer level, she must cut down her intake of alcoholic beverages. Lucy should drink no more than two drinks twice a week (four drinks total).

Recommended Diet

BREAKFAST IN COFFEE SHOP

1 scrambled egg on English muffin or whole-wheat toast with 1 tsp margarine

This sandwich is much lower in fat than the bacon/eggs/butter combination. However, Lucy should restrict her intake of high-cholesterol eggs to no more than two a week.

Tea with milk (low-fat if available)
2 tsp sugar

ALTERNATIVE BREAKFAST FOR EGGLESS DAYS

1 bowl hot cereal
2 slices whole-wheat toast or 1 toasted English muffin
1 pat margarine and/or 1 tsp jelly or jam

MIDMORNING SNACK

4–8 oz juice

But if she has to have her candy fix, she should have 5 chocolate kisses, which contain 125 calories, instead of the M&Ms, which weigh in at 240 calories.

1 cup low-fat milk

She could also eat yogurt mixed with fresh fruit. One or the other is necessary because she has to increase her calcium intake.

LUNCH AT RESTAURANT

1 slice pizza, blot excess oil with napkin

8 oz diet soda or seltzer with lemon

Seltzer is preferable because it contains no chemicals or sodium.

or

4 oz real soda with a lot of extra ice, no refills

Small box of raisins carried from home

These provide fiber and iron and taste good too!

DINNER

2 chicken or turkey franks (95% fat-free) made without skin with 1 tsp low-sodium mustard

2 buns (no butter or margarine)

4 oz seltzer mixed with 4 oz orange juice with pulp

1 fresh peach with skin

Fresh peaches are lower in calories than canned ones and are higher in fiber and better tasting too.

EVENING SNACK

1 cup skim milk with 1 tsp chocolate Ovaltine

It adds only 20 calories but lots of flavor.

1 low-calorie beer

Six Months Later

By following our simple suggestions, Lucy has made substantial changes in her eating and drinking style. She has dramatically reduced her intake of alcoholic beverages on her own, and in general she is doing a lot better. Lucy has rediscovered the joys of swimming, and manages to swim laps at her local "Y" two to three nights a week, which she feels has provided a good outlet for stress. Although she is never going to win any awards from *Prevention* magazine, Lucy has substantially reduced her consumption of saturated fats and has managed to reduce her triglycerides to 220 and her cholesterol to 235. Her HDL is up to 45, a modest but beneficial gain. In addition, she has lost 12 pounds, which has made a big improvement in her appearance.

What Their Experiences Mean to You

Lucy and Shelley learned a great deal about their eating patterns and their lifestyles simply by monitoring what they ate every day. Shelley saw that her "well-balanced" diet was too heavy in meat and lacking in fiber. Lucy saw that her frequent snacking on high-fat foods and nightly cocktails were the probable cause of her elevated triglycerides and cholesterol—not to mention her elevated weight. Once they were aware of their problems, they were able to do something about them.

There's an important lesson to learn from their experiences. Developing good eating habits is often as simple as taking a moment or two to reflect on what you're eating before it disappears into your mouth. In short, think before you eat. Ask yourself if you're making a wise choice. If you know that you're not, then ask yourself if it's possible to find a palatable substitution. The transition from a high-calorie cola to a fruit-flavored seltzer, or from a high-fat premium ice cream to a low-fat frozen yogurt is really not that difficult. In some cases, your taste buds may have to adjust, but within a short time the right choices will become the preferred choices.

HEART-HEALTHY AT A GLANCE

3,500 extra calories = 1 lb of body fat
1 gram of fat = 9 calories
1 gram of protein or carbohydrate = 4 calories

Eat no more than 30% of your daily calories in the form of any kind of fat. (1,800 calories; no more than 540 calories of fat).
Avoid saturated fats (raises cholesterol): no more than 10% of total calories.
Sparingly use polyunsaturated fats (lowers total cholesterol); no more than 10% of total calories.
Use monounsaturated fats (cuts LDL, not HDL); 10–15% of total calories.

IDEAL DIET RECOMMENDED BY THE AMERICAN HEART ASSOCIATION

25–30% fat
12–20% protein
50–63% carbohydrates

LEARNING TO MAINTAIN A NORMAL WEIGHT

Learning to make the right choices is the only way to maintain a normal weight. Chronic dieting—going from one crash diet to another—is not. We all know people who are constantly dieting, yet never seem to keep the weight off for any length of time. They shed pounds rapidly in the beginning, but quickly put them back. It is the "yo-yo" syndrome, also called weight cycling, and it may affect as many as 90 percent of all chronic dieters.

For dieters, the yo-yo syndrome is not only embarrassing and discouraging but it is an assault on the heart. Excess body weight is very stressful. For example, let's say a woman who should normally weigh 125 pounds shoots up to 200 pounds, and as a result she develops high blood pressure. Now her heart not only has to pump blood throughout 200 pounds of body tissue but it must do so against an increased pressure. The heart responds to the change in weight and pressure by producing certain proteins to help it pump harder and more efficiently.

This same woman goes on a severely restrictive, low-calorie diet and sheds 75 pounds in three months. Her blood pressure returns to normal and her body mass shrinks. Her heart no longer has to compensate for the high pressure and the added weight. But when she goes off the punishing diet—as most women do—she begins to gain weight all over again: first 10 pounds, then 20 pounds, until finally she weighs more than 200 pounds. To make matters worse, her blood pressure soars to new heights. Once again, her heart has to make drastic changes to accommodate the change in her body.

This same cycle is repeated over and over and over again, and each time her heart must rise to the challenge. As a result, her heart is never in a stable situation—it is always in a state of flux. It will continue to function until the strain becomes too great, or until it encounters an added stress that it cannot accommodate—the proverbial straw that breaks the camel's back.

If you want to lose weight safely and keep it off permanently, it must be done very gradually—no more than 2 pounds per week for as long as it takes and under the supervision of a qualified nutritional counselor. In addition, women with specific risk factors, such as diabetes and hypertension, should get professional advice because they may require special diets.

Genetics also play a major role in the pattern of weight gain over a lifetime.

If your parents are on the heavy side—even if you carefully watch every morsel that goes into your mouth—you may have a tendency to gain weight easily. It doesn't mean that your body won't look good, or that you won't be as healthy as the child of two superlean parents. But it does mean that you have to set realistic goals for yourself.

On the Metropolitan Life Insurance chart for recommended weight based on age and height there is a 30-pound range for the same specifications, depending on body build. If your family is heavier than average, unless you literally starve yourself, you will probably be on the high end of normal. If this is the case, it would be futile for you to try to diet down to the low end. As long as you're healthy at the heavier but normal weight, leave well enough alone. If you want to look trimmer, your best bet is to do muscle-tightening exercises for a sleeker line.

If you were overweight as a child, it may be even more difficult for you to maintain a normal weight as an adult. Although your body has the capacity to produce fat cells at any age, it goes into peak production between ages five and eleven, producing extra fat cells to accommodate the growth spurts typical of those formative years. If a child takes in the appropriate amount of calories, she will produce enough cells to accommodate growth without gaining excessive weight. If she takes in too many calories, she will manufacture extra fat cells. No matter how much she diets later in life, those cells will stay with her forever.

If she eats more food than she expends in energy, she will gain weight very rapidly because the existing fat cells can swell up to three times their usual size, resulting in obesity and the formation of even more fat cells. If she loses weight, they can shrink back to normal, but if she begins to take in more calories than she needs, the cells will once again expand and may even multiply. Thus, pediatricians are justifiably concerned about childhood obesity because of its possible effect on the child's immediate physical and emotional well-being, and because of its serious ramifications later in life.

BECOME AN EDUCATED CONSUMER

An educated nutritional consumer is not going to fall prey to fad diets or get-thin-quick schemes. She will make it her business to maintain a normal weight by eating a normal, well-balanced diet. In order to become an educated consumer, you have to keep up with the latest information on nutrition, which is no easy task. The field is rapidly changing. Practically every day, there are new findings being published in scientific journals about the relationship between nutrition and disease. Although it's impossible to read every article, you can stay abreast of these recent breakthroughs by subscribing to newsletters such as *Environmental Nutrition*, or the *Tufts University Diet and Nutrition Letter*, two excellent publications that are used by professionals as well as laymen. The American Heart Association and the American Dietetic Association also provide good, easy-to-understand information on nutrition. In addition, a trip to the local branch of the Government Printing Office can yield a goldmine in terms of brochures and pamphlets on food.

During the past decade, we have gained a great deal of knowledge about the relationship between diet and CAD. We are fortunate in that we are the first generation of women who are able to take full advantage of this knowledge. In many cases, we can prevent the onset of disease by eating sensibly and taking good care of ourselves. However, good health is not always easy to achieve. Eating properly does take more thought and preparation than grabbing whatever happens to be around. If you're busy to begin with, the thought of adding more responsibility to your packed day may be daunting. But think of it this way. You were born with one heart that must last you for a lifetime. Whatever you can do to keep it strong and functioning well is worth the effort.

RESOURCES: See page 235.

VIII

IT'S ONLY
THE BEGINNING

❧

EPILOGUE

The Female Heart may be one of the first books ever written on women and heart disease, but I am confident that it will not be the last. Although we now know a great deal more about the development and course of CAD than we did a decade ago, we still have a great deal more to learn.

There are many questions about heart disease that are unanswered, especially when it comes to women and children: What roles do hormones play in protecting women against CAD? Is estrogen replacement therapy (ERT) worth the risk? Should all children eat a low-fat diet? Do women need to be as concerned about cholesterol as men? Which cholesterol-lowering drugs work best for women? Which cardiac medications work best for women? These are just some of the issues that require and deserve further exploration.

Unfortunately, many of these questions are likely to remain a mystery because basic medical research is so chronically underfunded in the United States. The budget of the National Institutes of Health, which pays for virtually all of the medical research that is done in this country, has not kept pace with the national need for better healthcare. It is becoming increasingly difficult for even the most talented young scientists to get money to support their work. As a result, important ideas that have the potential to save lives and improve the quality of life for millions of people are not being explored.

Funding basic medical research is not welfare nor is it charity. These dedicated researchers work very hard for very little money. From society's point of view, the return on the investment is great. For example, in the 1960s and 1970s, NIH-funded scientists discovered how DNA could be cut and manipulated by using enzymes found in bacteria—a technology now commonly known as genetic engineering. This is a prime example of how apparently esoteric research can directly pave the way for enormous advances in how well we can care for patients. This research has also shown us how to produce synthetic hormones and will perhaps even produce a vaccine for AIDS. The tragedy is that in today's climate this type of innovative research would be considered "pie in the sky" by Congress who might well dismiss it as irrelevant to the problems of public health. As the NIH rejects more and more applications for research grants, more and more dedicated scientists are leaving the profession to pursue other more financially rewarding endeavors. Their departure is an irreversible blow to our healthcare system and one that patients will pay for dearly within a short time.

We are already paying for the CAD epidemic financially and emotionally. In direct healthcare costs alone, Americans dole out 8 billion dollars annually to pay for this disease. Another 60 billion dollars is stripped from the economy each year in terms of unemployment, reduced worker productivity, disability, and other hidden costs of heart disease. Money is not the only issue. Tens of millions of families are actively caring for and supporting relatives with heart disease. It just makes good economic sense to devote substantial resources to the number-one killer of both men and women.

It is critical that the people who do get money for research devote some of their time to the needs of women and children. It is obvious that these two groups have been neglected for many years. As women—and as human beings—we must all assume the task of making sure that children are being treated fairly and that their health needs are not being ignored. With neither economic nor political power, children are the weak link in our society and in need of a strong advocate.

We also have a responsibility to maintain our own health. Since the surgeon general first called attention to the dangers of smoking in 1964, study after study has confirmed the toxic effect of smoking on our bodies. Yet millions of women still smoke and millions of teenage girls still believe that this lethal habit will make them sophisticated and attractive. Millions of other women turn to smoking as a means of coping with stress and frustration. When I challenge them in my office, they see stopping as yet another deprivation. In fact, I am only trying to save their lives.

Finally, we as women—the caregivers of society—must learn to take better care of ourselves. Of course we get a great deal of pleasure and fulfillment from caring for our families. Most of us cherish that part of our lives and would not give it up for anything in the world. But it is not useful for either ourselves or our families if we always put our needs last. We cannot care for others until we care for ourselves.

RESOURCES

Chapter 3: Synthetic Hormones and the Heart

For information on estrogen replacement therapy, contact:

National Women's Health Center
1325 G Street, NW
Washington, DC 20005

American College of Obstetricians and Gynecologists
409 12th Street, SW
Washington, DC 20024–2188
Tel. 202/638–5577

Chapter 7: Cardiac Arrhythmia

For a list of hospitals with electrophysiology units, or for a list of specialists in your area, contact:

North American Society for Pacing and Electrophysiology
13 Eaton Court
Wellesley Hills, MA 02181

For information on obtaining a Medic Alert bracelet, contact:

Medic Alert Foundation
475 Fifth Avenue
New York, NY 10017

Chapter 13: A Lethal Dose of Stress

To find a specialist in treating addictions, contact:

The American Society of Addiction Medicine
12 W. 21st Street
New York, NY 10010
Tel. 212/206–6770

To find support groups, contact:

Alcoholics Anonymous
Check local telephone directory under "A" for nearest group

Al-Anon
1327 Broadway
New York, NY 10018
Tel. 212/302–7240

Cocaine Anonymous Hotline
To locate the group nearest you, call:
800/437–8998

For assistance in quitting smoking, contact:

Smokenders
This international group provides workshops for the public and at the workplace.
For information about their six-week program, call:
Tel. 800/828–4357

American Lung Association
This group has local chapters nationwide that sponsor the Freedom from Smoking
Program that includes workshops and audio and video cassettes for home use.
Special programs are geared for pregnant women, families, and individuals. For
information, check with your local Lung Association chapter or call:
Tel. 212/315–8700

Chapter 16: The Road to Recovery

For information on cardiac support groups, contact:

Mended Hearts
7320 Greenville Avenue
Dallas, TX 75231
Tel. 214/706–1340

Chapter 17: Working with Your Doctor

For a list of board-certified internists, contact:

American Society of Internal Medicine
1101 Vermont Avenue, NW
Washington, DC 20005
202/289–1700

To request an AMA physician profile, contact:

American Medical Association
535 North Dearborn Street
Chicago, IL 60610

Chapter 18: Good News for Women About Exercise

For information on how to select a health club or an exercise trainer, contact:

American College of Sports Medicine
P.O. Box 1440
Indianapolis, IN 46206
Attn: Certification Department, Certification for Health and Fitness Professionals

Chapter 19: A Woman's Diet and Heart Disease

For information on nutritional counseling, contact:

The American Dietetic Association
216 W. Jackson
Suite 800
Chicago, IL 60606
Tel. 312/899–0040

For information on current nutrition news, subscribe to the following newsletters:

Tufts University Diet and Nutrition Letter
P.O. Box 857
Boulder, CO 80322
800/274–7581

Environmental Nutrition
2112 Broadway
Suite 200
New York, NY 10023

For information on diabetes, contact:

American Diabetes Association
1660 Duke Street
Alexandria, VA 22314

SELECTED BIBLIOGRAPHY

Abbott, R. D., et al. "High Density Lipoprotein Cholesterol, Total Cholesterol Screening, and Myocardial Infarction. The Framingham Study." *Arteriosclerosis* 8:207–211, 1988.

American Heart Association: "Silent Epidemic: The Truth About Women & Heart Disease." Dallas, Texas.

Barnett, R. C., L. Biener, and G. K. Baruch (eds). *Gender & Stress.* New York: The Free Press, 1987.

Barzel, U. S. "Estrogens in the Prevention and Treatment of Postmenopausal Osteoporosis: A Review." *American Journal of Medicine* 85:847–850, 1988.

Benigni, A., G. Gregorini, T. Frusca, et al. "Effect of Low-Dose Aspirin on Fetal and Maternal Generation of Thromboxane by Platelets in Women at Risk for Pregnancy-Induced Hypertension." *New England Journal of Medicine* 321:357–362, 1989.

Bergkvist, L., H. O. Adami, I. Persson, et al. "The Risk of Breast Cancer and Estrogen-Progestin Replacement." *New England Journal of Medicine* 321:293–297, 1989.

Blair, S., H. Kohl, R. Pappenbarger, et al. "Physical Fitness and All-Cause Mortality: A Prospective Study of Healthy Men and Women." *Journal of the American Medical Association* 262:2395–2401, 1989.

Blakeslee, Sandra. "Study Hints of Harm in Heart Operations." *New York Times,* February 29, 1990.

Blaufox, M. "Systemic Arterial Hypertension in Pediatric Practice." *Pediatric Clinics of North America,* 18(2); 577–593, 1971.

Braunwald, E., ed. *A Textbook of Cardiovascular Medicine,* 3rd ed. Philadelphia: W. B. Saunders, 1988.

Buchwald, H., R. Varco, John Matts, et al. "Effect of Partial Ileal Bypass Surgery on Mortality and Morbidity from Coronary Heart Disease in Patients with Hypercholesterolemia." *New England Journal of Medicine* 323:946–954, 1990.

Bush, T. L., L. D. Cowen, E. Barrett-Conner, et al. "Estrogen Use and All-Cause Mortality: Preliminary Results from the Lipid Research Clinics Follow-up Study." *Journal of the American Medical Association* 249:903–906, 1983.

Castelli, W. P. "Epidemiology of Coronary Heart Disease: The Framingham Study. I. Methods and Risk Factors." *American Journal of Medicine* 76:4–12, 1984.

Castelli, W. P. "The Triglyceride Issue: A View from Framingham." *American Heart Journal* 112:432–437, 1986.

Centerall, B. S. "Premenopausal Hysterectomy and Cardiovascular Disease." *American Journal of Obstetrics and Gynecology* 139:58–61, 1981.

Chesney, M. A., and R. H. Rosenman. *Anger and Hostility in Cardiovascular and Behavioral Disorders*. Washington: Hemisphere Publishing Corporation, 1985.

Clapp, J. F., et al. "Maternal Physiologic Adaptations to Early Human Pregnancy." *American Journal of Obstetrics and Gynecology* 159:1456–1460, 1988.

Clark, S. I. "Labor and Delivery in the Patient with Structural Cardiac Disease." *Clinical Perinatology* 12:695–703, 1986.

"Committee on Atherosclerosis and Hypertension in Childhood of the Council on Cardiovascular Disease in the Young and the Nutrition Committee, American Heart Association: Diagnosis and Treatment of Primary Hyperlipidemia in Childhood. Position Statement." *Circulation* 74:1181–1188, 1986.

Detre, T., et al. "Management of the Menopause." *Annals of Internal Medicine* 88:373–378, 1978.

Dukakis, K., and J. Scovell. *Now You Know*. New York: Simon and Schuster Inc., 1990.

Eaker, Ed, et al. "Spouse Behavior and Coronary Heart Disease in Men: Prospective Results from the Framingham Study. II: Modification of Risk in Type A Husbands According to the Social and Psychological Status of Their Wives." *American Journal of Epidemiology* 118:23–41, 1983.

Eaker, E., B. Packard, N. Wenger, et al. (eds.). *Coronary Heart Disease in Women*. New York: Haymarket-Doyma, Inc., 1987.

Egan, B., and A. Weder. "Deleterious Effects of NaCl Restriction." Paper delivered at the American Heart Association, 62d Scientific Session, 1989.

Ehsani, A. A. "Cardiac Rehabilitation." *Cardiology Clinics* 2:63–69, 1984.

Evans, G. L., et al. "Pulmonary Embolism During Pregnancy." *Journal of the American Medical Association* 206:320–326, 1968.

Friedman, M., and R. H. Rosenman. *Type A Behavior and Your Heart*. New York: Fawcett Crest, 1974.

Gastel, B., et al. "Estrogen Use and Postmenopausal Women: A Basis for Informed Decisions. NIH Consensus Development." *Journal of Family Practice* 11:1151–1160, 1980.

Gianopoulos, J. G. "Cardiac Disease in Pregnancy." *Medical Clinics of North America* 73:639–651, 1989.

Gilligan, C. *In a Different Voice: Psychological Theory and Women's Development*. Cambridge, Massachusetts, and London: Harvard University Press, 1982.

Glick, I. D., and S. E. Bennet. "Psychiatric Complications of Progesterone and Oral Contraceptives." *Journal of Clinical Psychopharmacology* 1(6):350–367, 1981.

Gordon T., and W. B. Kannel. "Drinking Habits and Cardiovascular Disease: The Framingham Study." *American Heart Journal* 105:667–673, 1983.

Gordon T., et al. "High Density Lipoprotein as a Protective Factor Against Coronary Heart Disease. The Framingham Study." *American Journal of Public Health* 62:707–714, 1977.

Gordon, T., et al. "Diabetes, Blood Lipids, and the Role of Obesity in Coronary Heart Disease Risk for Women. The Framingham Study." *Annals of Internal Medicine* 87:393–397, 1977.

Gotto, A., J. La Rosa, et al. "The Cholesterol Facts: A Summary of the Evidence Relating Dietary Fats, Blood Cholesterol, and Coronary Artery Disease. Commissioned by the Task Force on Cholesterol Issues of the American Heart Association." 1989.

Guidelines for Exercise Testing and Prescription. American College of Sports Medicine, 3rd ed., Lea and Febiger, Philadelphia, 1986.

Hankins, G. D., et al. "Myocardial Infarction During Pregnancy. A Review." *American Journal of Obstetrics and Gynecology* 65:139–46, 1985.

Harvey, R., E. Doyle, K. Ellis, et al. *Nomenclature and Criteria for Diagnosis of Diseases of the Heart and Great Vessels* (The Criteria Committee of the New York Heart Association), 7th ed. Little, Brown and Company, Boston, 1973.

Hastreiter, A., et al. "The Electrocardiogram in the Newborn Period. 1. The Normal Infant." *Journal of Pediatrics* 78:146–56, 1971.

Haynes, S. G., and M. Feinleib. "Woman, Work, and Coronary Heart Disease: Prospective Findings from the Framingham Heart Study." *American Journal of Public Health* 70:133–41, 1980.

Haynes, S. G., et al. "Spouse Behavior and Coronary Heart Disease in Men: Prospective Results from the Framingham Heart Study. I. Concordance of Risk Factors and the Relationship of Psychosocial Status to Coronary Incidence." *American Journal of Epidemiology* 118:1–22, 1983.

Haynes, S. G., et al. "The Relationship of Psychosocial Factors to Coronary Heart Disease from the Framingham Study. I. Methods and Risk Factors." *American Journal of Epidemiology* 118:1–22, 1983.

Higgins, M., et al. "Hazards of Obesity: the Framingham Experience." *Acta Medical Scandanavian Supplement* 723:23–36, 1988.

Homans, D. C. "Peripartum Cardiomyopathy." *New England Journal of Medicine* 312:1432–1437, 1985.

Johnson, T. "The Cholesterol Controversy." *Harvard Medical Letter* 15:1–3, 1989.

Kannel, W. B. "Habitual Level of Physical Activity and Risk of Coronary Heart Disease: The Framingham Study." *Canadian Medical Association Journal* 96:811–812, 1967.

Kannel, W. B. "Metabolic Risk Factors for Coronary Heart Disease in Women: Perspective from the Framingham Study." *American Heart Journal* 114:413–419, 1987.

Kannel, W. B., et al. "Fibrinogen, Cigarette Smoking and Risk of Cardiovascular Disease: Insights from the Framingham Study." *American Heart Journal* 113:1006–1010, 1987.

Kannel, W. B., et al. "Cardiac Failure and Sudden Death in the Framingham Study." *American Heart Journal* 115:869–875, 1988.

Kannel, W. B., et al. "A General Cardiovascular Risk Profile: The Framingham Study." *American Journal of Cardiology* 38:46–51, 1976.

Kannel, W. B., et al. "Menopause and Risk of Cardiovascular Disease: The Framingham Study." *Annals of Internal Medicine* 85:447–452, 1976.

Kannel, W. B., et al. "Systolic Versus Diastolic Blood Pressure and Risk of Coronary Heart Disease: The Framingham Study." *American Journal of Cardiology* 27:335–346, 1971.

Kavanaugh, T. "Distance Running and Cardiac Rehabilitation: Physiologic and Psychosocial Considerations." *Clinical Sports Medicine* 3:513–526, 1984.

Khan, S., S. Nessim, R. Gray, et al. "Increased Mortality of Women in Coronary Artery Bypass Surgery: Evidence for Referral Bias." *Annals of Internal Medicine* 112:561–567, 1990.

Kilcoyne, M. "Adolescent Hypertension." *American Journal of Medicine* 58:735–739, 1975.

Knopp, R. H. "Cardiovascular Effects of Endogenous and Exogenous Sex Hormones over a Woman's Lifetime." *American Journal of Obstetrics and Gynecology* 158:1630–1643, 1988.

Korenman, S. G. "Menopausal Endocrinology and Management." *Archives of Internal Medicine* 142:1131–1136, 1982.

Lapidus, L., et al. "Menopausal Age and Risk of Cardiovascular Disease and Death: A 12 Year Follow-up of Participants in the Population Study of Women in Gothenberg, Sweden." *Acta Obstetrical Journal* (supplement) 130:37–41, 1985.

Leaf, D. A. "Exercise During Pregnancy. Guidelines and Controversies." *Postgraduate Medicine* 85:233–234, 1989.

Legato, M. (ed.). *The Developing Heart. Clinical Implications of Its Molecular Biology and Physiology.* Boston: Martinus Nijhoff, 1984.

Legato, M. *The Myocardial Cell for the Clinical Cardiologist.* Mt. Kisco, New York: Futura Publishing Company, Inc., 1973.

Legato, M. (ed.). *The Stressed Heart.* Boston: Martinus Nijhoff, 1987.

Lerner, D. J., and W. B. Kannel. "Patterns of Coronary Heart Disease Morbidity and Mortality in the Sexes: A 26 Year Follow-up of the Framingham Population." *American Journal of Cardiology* 111:383–390, 1986.

Lindheimer, M., et al. "Preeclampsia: Pathophysiology, Diagnosis, and Management." *Annual Review of Medicine* 40:233–250, 1989.

Manson, J., G. Colditz, M. Stampfer, et al. "A Prospective Study of Obesity and Risk of Coronary Heart Disease in Women." *New England Journal of Medicine* 322:882–889, 1990.

Mashini, I. S. "Serial Noninvasive Evaluation of Cardiovascular Hemodynamics During Pregnancy." *American Journal of Obstetrics and Gynecology* 156:1208–1213, 1987.

Masserlie, F. H., et al. "Disparate Cardiovascular Findings in Men and Women with Essential Hypertension." *Annals of Internal Medicine* 107:158–61, 1987.

Matthews, K. A., et al. "Menopause and Risk Factors for Coronary Heart Disease." *New England Journal of Medicine* 321:641–646, 1989.

Morrow, R. J., et al. "Fetal and Maternal Hemodynamic Responses to Exercise in Pregnancy Assessed by Doppler Ultrasonography." *American Journal of Obstetrics and Gynecology* 160:138–140, 1989.

Morton, M. J., et al. "Exercise Dynamics in Late Gestation: Effects of Physical Training." *American Journal of Obstetrics and Gynecology* 152:91–97, 1985.

"1990 Report on Special Programming for Women: A Position Paper on Women's Alcoholism Treatment." New York State Division of Alcoholism and Alcohol Abuse.

Nachtigall, L., and J. Heilman. *Estrogen: The Facts Can Change Your Life.* Los Angeles: The Body Press, 1986.

National Heart Lung and Blood Institute Workshop, October 1988. "Recommendations Regarding Public Screening for Measuring Blood Cholesterol." *Archives of Internal Medicine* 149:2650–2654, 1989.

Nora, J. "Identifying the Child at Risk for Coronary Disease As an Adult: A Strategy for Prevention." *Journal of Pediatrics* 97:706–714, 1980.

Ornish, Dean. *Dr. Dean Ornish's Program for Reversing Heart Disease.* Random House, New York, 1990.

Pollock, M. L., and A. E. Pels. "Exercise Prescription for the Cardiac Patient: An Update." *Clinical Sports Medicine* 3:425–442, 1984.

Raymond, R., et al. "Cardiovascular Problems During Pregnancy." *Cleveland Clinics Journal of Medicine* 19:37–56, 1987.

Reeves, J., A. Oberman, W. Jones, et al. *American Journal of Cardiology* 33:423–430, 1974.

Rothfelder, J. *Heart Rhythms: Breakthrough Treatments for Cardiac Arrhythmia—The Silent Killer of 400,000 Americans Each Year.* Little, Brown & Co., Boston, 1989.

Roy, C., and N. Galeano. "Childhood Antecedents of Adult Degenerative Disease." *Pediatric Clinics of North America* 32:517–533, 1985.

Sarrel, P. M. "Sexuality in the Middle Years." *Obstetrical Gynecological Clinics of North America* 14:49–62, 1987.

Savaroni, I., et al. "Risk Factors for Coronary Artery Disease in Healthy Persons with Hyperinsulinemia and Normal Glucose Tolerance." *New England Journal of Medicine* 320:702–706, 1989.

Schatzkin, A., et al. "The Epidemiology of Sudden Unexpected Death: Risk Factors for Men and Women in the Framingham Heart Study." *American Heart Journal* 107:1300–1306, 1984.

Schatzkin, A., et al. "Sudden Death in the Framingham Heart Study. Differences in Incidence and Risk Factors by Sex and Coronary Disease Status." *American Journal of Epidemiology* 120:888–890, 1984.

Schiff, E., E. Peleg, M. Goldenberg, et al. "The Use of Aspirin to Prevent Pregnancy-Induced Hypertension and Lower the Ratio of Thromboxane A_2 to Prostacyclin in Relatively High Risk Pregnancies." *New England Journal of Medicine* 321:351–356, 1989.

Semchyshyn, S., and C. Colman. *How to Prevent Miscarriage and Other Crises of Pregnancy.* New York: Macmillan, 1989.

Silfverstolpe, G., and N. Crona. "Hormonal Replacement Therapy—Cardiovascular Disease." *Acta Obstetrical Gynecology Scandinavia* (supplement) 134:93–95, 1986.

Silver, H. M. "Acute Hypertensive Crises in Pregnancy." *Medical Clinics of North America* 73:623–638, 1989.

The Surgeon General's Report on Nutrition and Health. Rocklin, Califorhia: Prima Publishing and Communications, 1988.

Stadel, B. V. "Oral Contraceptives and Cardiovascular Disease" (two parts). *Bulletin of New York Academy of Medicine* 305:612–618, 672–677, 1981.

Texon, M. "Guest Editorial: The Cholesterol–Heart Disease Hypothesis (Critique)— Time to Change the Course?" *Bulletin of the New York Academy of Medicine* 65:836–841, 1989.

Tobin, J., S. Wassertheil-Smoller, J. Wexler, et al. "Sex Bias in Considering Coronary Bypass Surgery." *Annals of Internal Medicine* 107:19–24, 1987.

Tyroler, H. A. "Cholesterol and Cardiovascular Disease. An Overview of the Lipid Research Clinics (LRC) Epidemiologic Studies as Background for the LRC Primary Prevention Trial." *American Journal of Cardiology* 54:14C–19C, 1984.

Veille, J. C., et al. "Cardiac Size and Function in Pregnancy-Induced Hypertension." *American Journal of Obstetrics and Gynecology* 1:443–449, 1984.

Walter, H. J., et al. "Modification of Risk Factors for Coronary Heart Disease: Five Year Results of a School-based Interventional Trial." *New England Journal of Medicine* 318:1093–1099, 1988.

Weidman, W., P. Kwiterovich, Jr., et al. "Diagnosis and Treatment of Primary Hyperlipidemia in Childhood: A Joint Statement for Physicians by the Committee on Atherosclerosis and Hypertension in Childhood of the Council on Cardiovascular Disease in the Young and the Nutrition Committee, American Heart Association." *Circulation* 74:5.2, 1986.

White, M., R. Yeater, R. B. Martin, et al. "Effects of Aerobic Dancing and Walking on Cardiovascular Function and Muscular Strength in Postmenopausal Women." *Journal of Sports Medicine* pp. 159–167, 1984.

Williams, G., B. Grant, et al. "Population Projections Using DSM-II Criteria: Alcohol Abuse and Dependence, 1990–2000." *Epidemiologic Bulletin* No. 23, *Alcohol Health & Research World* 13:366–377, 1989.

Wilson, P. W., et al. "Coronary Risk Prediction in Adults (the Framingham Heart Study)." *American Journal of Cardiology* 59:91–94, 1987.

INDEX